Healing the Pain of Pet Loss
Letters in Memoriam

Edited by

Kymberly Smith

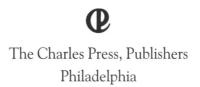

The Charles Press, Publishers
Philadelphia

For My Paul

Copyright © 1998 by The Charles Press, Publishers, Inc.

All rights reserved

This publication may not be reproduced in whole or in part, or stored in a retrieval system, or transmitted in any form or by any means — electronic, mechanical, photocopying, scanning, recording or otherwise — without consent in writing from The Charles Press, Publishers.

The Charles Press, Publishers
Post Office Box 15715
Philadelphia, PA 19103
(215) 545-8933 Telephone
(215) 545-8937 Telefax
ChsPrsPub@aol.com

Library of Congress Cataloging-in-Publication Data

Healing the pain of pet loss: letters in memoriam / edited by Kymberly Smith.
p. cm.
Includes bibliographical references.
ISBN 0-914783-79-3
1. Pet owners — Psychology. 2. Pets — Death — Psychological aspects. 3. Bereavement — Psychological aspects. 4. Pet owners — Correspondence.
5. Bereavement — Personal narratives.
I. Smith, Kymberly.
SF411.47.M9 1996
155.9'37 — DC20
96-28496

Printed in the United States of America

ISBN 0-914783-79-3

Acknowledgments

I am indebted to the following people for their helpful information: Roberta Kalechofsky of Jews for Animal Rights; Joan Clair, Director of Ministries for Animals; and Frances Arnetta of Christians Helping Animals and People, Inc.

My very special thanks to Lisa Sheets, editor of *I Love Cats* magazine, and the editors of *Dog Fancy* magazine for printing my requests for letters.

My deepest gratitude to Lauren Meltzer of The Charles Press, Publishers for making it possible for this book to reach others. And, finally, a personal note of appreciation to Elizabeth Dornberger for all her hard work and encouragement, and for always believing in friendship.

Preface

The idea for this book came about in much the same way many things do in life — I desperately needed something I could not find. I was trying to come to terms with the sudden disappearance of my beloved cat, Gusser, and at the same time, I was faced with the impending death of my other cherished cat, Seeya. To make matters worse, I thought no one understood the intensity of the pain I was experiencing. I didn't know how or where I would find the emotional strength to deal with the heartache of Seeya's death, especially because I hadn't yet managed to find a way to cope with the loss of Gusser.

Finding limited solace in my friends and family, I started looking for books on pet loss and bereavement, hoping that they might give me some advice or consolation. But, to my surprise, I couldn't find a single book that *really* helped me, one that offered me the kind of comfort and support I wanted. Most of them were too clinical in their approach and too theoretical; feelings and stages of grief were identified, categorized and analyzed, but that was not information that would help me heal and feel better. Moreover, they were mostly discussions of and theories on *other* people's losses; they were sorely lacking in subjective accounts from people who had actually had firsthand experience with the kind of severe loss that I was now experiencing. Because I just couldn't seem to find a book that contained this kind of information, I decided that I would try to write my own book, one that would *really* help people who, like me, were suffering from the loss of their animal friend.

I soon realized that this was an inflated idea, much easier to plan than to execute. I really had no idea what I could put in my book that would make it unique and truly help people who were in pain. Then I came up with the idea of contacting others who were in the same situation — who had also experienced the pain of losing an animal companion. I figured that they knew *firsthand* about this kind of pain. From them I knew I could get helpful and honest material for my book

I began by sending a few letters to the editorial sections of magazines for animal lovers, asking readers to send me their stories about losing their animal companions. My family and friends thought my search would yield only sparse returns, and truthfully, so did I. Never did I anticipate the hundreds of letters that soon began filling my post office box. They came from men, women and children. Some of them were from therapists, editors, nurses and teachers. Others were written by police officers, veterans and unemployed persons. Most were from America, but some came from other countries. Some were over 20 pages long, and several included photos of their animal friends.

At first, I wondered why all these people were willing to share such a private piece of their souls with me — a complete stranger. But soon I understood. It seems that writing these letters provided these people with a much-needed release of emotion and an opportunity to speak freely and lovingly of their animal friends. It was cathartic for them in a way that I had never anticipated. Most of the letter writers made it clear that finding someone with a sympathetic ear was nearly impossible because their loss concerned an animal. Even though awareness of the intensity of this kind of grief is increasing, there are many people, including professional therapists, who think that the loss of a pet is no big deal. As a result, many people keep their feelings to themselves, making an already horrible situation even worse.

Initially, when I asked for these stories, I had planned to use the information in them as research. I never dreamed that I would be given such deeply personal insights into the lives and hearts of people I didn't know. I was simply overwhelmed by the depth of emotion and pain and love expressed in the letters. I knew I had to change my plans for my book because nothing I could write *about* these letters would be as powerful as the letters themselves. I realized that the best way to pass on this wonderful gift that had been so helpful and healing to me was to offer the letters for others to read — keeping them as close to the original as possible.

In ways that I never anticipated, the letters turned out to be healing to me. They comforted me, gave me support and understanding and made me realize that there were many other people in the world who felt the same way I did. I was not alone, and as long as I had these beautiful and compassionate letters to read, I would never again have to feel isolated in my grief. In the same way, I hope you, the reader, will feel a comforting and supportive companionship with the letter writers — these are people who know how it feels. I like to think of the book as a portable and personal support group that you can pull out and read any time you may need it. You will be able to read how other people felt and reacted to their loss, how they solved their problems and coped — and in some cases, how they didn't.

Hopefully, you will find a letter in the book that speaks to you personally, that will be important to you in one way or another. Whether a story moves you, makes you think about issues in your own life or prompts you to look at things in new and different ways, I believe that the stories will speak to each reader on a different level. I found one letter that did just that for me and I carry it with me always. I have included letters from many different types of people with many different types of grief reactions with the hope that every reader will be able to find something of personal meaning.

There are no words to express how much I owe to each and every one of you who wrote to me and how much you helped me in accepting my own losses. Although I can never thank you in person, I hope I can thank you in a different way — by passing on to others the very special gift you gave me. Space would not allow me to include all of the letters that I received and I apologize to those writers whose letters I was not able to include. Every single letter was beautiful and inspiring and I thank every one of you.

The lines of communication between the people who have

loved and lost a cherished animal friend are always open in this book. And, as I have found out myself, there is something extremely powerful that exists between people who are bonded in traumatic experience. We *can* help each other. As you make your journey through sorrow toward acceptance and healing, I hope you find empathy and reassurance in the pages of this book.

Kymberly Smith

Contents

We Were a Perfect Family   1

The life and death of an important family member are celebrated and shared by this family, their church and their friends.

Little Persons   7

A woman describes the terrible experience of losing *both* of her cherished pets within one week.

The Special Ones   12

A beautiful story of the relationship between a woman and her Doberman pinscher.

We Had a Bond   16

After the death of her cats, this woman feels pain and anger at everything and everyone, including God.

The Caregiver   23

Memories of a nurturing collie help a family cope with the pain after her death.

Not "Only a Dog" — 29

A young woman tells of the battle she and her dog waged before death took the life of her beloved companion.

When Part of Me Died — 33

Even though the sudden death of this young woman's dog haunts her with thoughts of suicide, she has found a way to keep going.

Beloved Friends — 40

A woman tells the story of the tragic and sudden death of her two horses.

My Furry Soulmate — 44

This writer describes how fortunate she was to have a good support system when her beloved companion died.

Tears for Joy, Tears for Sorrow — 47

An immigrant finds it hard to manage without her beloved cat who had helped her adjust to life in America.

I Am Not Comforted — 50

An amazing story about how a cat stopped a nurse from committing suicide.

The Cat Who Died for Me — 58

A woman is certain that her cat died of a broken heart.

A Mother Cat Mourns   61

This story shows that, like people, animals grieve and need comfort too.

Death by Negligence?   66

An emigrant from Romania describes the trauma she experienced with a veterinary hospital she thought she could trust.

Telepathy   70

Even though this older man believes he couldn't express the grief he felt when his cat died, he finds solace in one very special thought.

The Disappeared   74

A woman is conflicted with fear, guilt, hope and disappointment when her cat disappears without a trace.

My Feline Children   77

A man explains how losing a pet is just like losing a child; you cannot fill the place of one with another.

A Big, Empty Spot   80

A 12-year-old girl is afraid she might have caused the disappearance of her cat.

Puppyraisers   82

People who raise and train dogs to help the physically challenged are in a very difficult situation.

A Dog's Courage — 86

A woman with a serious disease learns some important lessons about courage from her German shepherd.

My Dearest Companion — 91

Because this writer depended so heavily on her dog, not only to protect her and love her, but also to act as her ears, the loneliness she feels upon his death is overwhelming.

My Buddy and Protector — 97

This husband and wife find a comforting way of dealing with the death of their beloved dog.

My Little Ferret Friend — 100

A woman gathers strength from knowing she did the right thing by her sick ferret.

A Naturally Centered Being — 104

A man learns, only after the death of his dog, how much he had depended on her.

My Little Lu Lu — 108

A young girl wonders whether her hopes for her cat's return mean that she is not facing up to facts.

Riding Max's Back — 111

A little girl thought that she caused her dog's death.

Swept Away   112

After losing her cat and virtually everything else she owned and held dear, this woman explains what she did to heal her heart.

How Love Can Hurt and Heal   116

The loss of his animal companions made this animal-loving deputy sheriff almost die from grief before a total coincidence put him back on the path of healing.

Tribute to a Gray Furry Friend   123

The writer explains how burial in a pet cemetery was helpful to this family after losing a dear rabbit friend.

Animals Are Better   126

A woman cannot find the support she needs after the death of her beloved animal friend.

My Closest and Best Friend   129

A teenager tries to deal with profound mourning after losing the dog that meant more to her than anything.

Love of the Wild   132

The death of an exotic animal teaches this woman many lessons about herself and other people.

Separation Blues   136

Angered and sad that her dog was taken away, a young woman vows that no one will take from her again.

"Mom, Gussie Died" — 140

How it feels to lose an animal friend after 21 years.

Bestest House Mouse Ever — 142

A woman tells a wonderful story about her companion mouse.

The Scales of Memory — 146

An incredible story about a precocious iguana and the unique way his owner dealt with his grief.

A Lady and a Fat Rabbit — 151

The joy these animals gave a family while living helps sustain them in dealing with their death.

Helping Children with Death — 156

A mother teaches her children about the love of animals and the pain of grief.

Appendix

The Spiritual Dimension	161
Introduction	161
Western Thoughts	163
Eastern Thoughts	171
The Humanist Perspective	176
Thoughts from the Letter Writers	178
Helpful Resources	184

Letters in Memoriam

We Were a Perfect Family

Dear Kymberly,

I was glad to see your letter in *Dog Fancy* magazine about a book on losing your animal because I have some ideas on the subject. For example, if you really love animals, you will feel as brokenhearted when your pet dies as you will when a relative or a dear human friend dies. People who don't have pets may think that people like us are fools or that we're just plain stupid for feeling this way, but they don't understand. It is so important for pet lovers to know that it is human to grieve over the loss of a pet and that there are many other people who feel this way. Loving a pet is wonderful and those who have never had the experience are really missing out.

    I've had many pets over the years but I want to tell you about one very special one — my black miniature poodle, Cinder. My mother gave him to me and my husband on the day after we returned from our honeymoon. We both fell in love with Cinder immediately. He was so cute and adorable and so tiny he fit in the palm of my hand. Being ever so young and just having left the security of his mother, he was afraid and needed love and attention.

When my husband and I went to work we would fence Cinder into the kitchen, but he always managed to get out. He would find his way into the bedroom and he'd go to sleep right next to my side of the bed. In about a month he was able to jump on the bed and he would sleep there for hours in total comfort. I did not chase him off because he was so content. When I would come home from work he would be so happy he would jump and squeal. I looked forward to seeing him every day. When we went to bed at night we'd put Cinder between us, just like a baby. He loved it and never moved all night. When it was cold, he slept under the covers with us and we would all cuddle.

Cinder showed us how much he loved us in different ways. My husband traveled a great deal back then and when he packed his suitcase, Cinder would show us that he didn't want my husband to leave by removing his socks from the suitcase. If we put the socks back, Cinder would take them out again. One time he got into the suitcase as if to say, Take me with you!

When I became pregnant with my first daughter, I quit my job and this made Cinder very happy. When I would lie on the couch for a nap or to watch TV, he would nuzzle next to my stomach and when he would feel the baby move, he would look up at me with such curiosity.

When I came home from the hospital after giving birth to my daughter, Cinder jumped all over me. We showed him our new addition and he was very curious and smelled her carefully. When we placed the baby in the bassinet, he climbed under it and from that day on, he slept there every night.

When someone other than my husband or I went near the baby, Cinder would growl until we assured him no harm would occur. I have to admit that I loved him just as much as I love my daughter.

Cinder always gave me comfort. I always spoke to him and he understood everything. This did not surprise me because when there is love of that magnitude anything is possible. When we were home he never left our sides; he was always there, always snuggling next to us, always near our daughter. I felt like I had the perfect family.

A few years later we had another child and Cinder acted the same as she had with our first daughter. Cinder slept in their room between their beds. The girls always played with him; they would even dress him up and put him in their baby doll carriage. And the best part was he always stayed put. He loved it. I don't know who acted more like a kid, my children or my dog.

My husband would walk Cinder before he went to work, when he returned and again late at night and Cinder loved these walks. We each had our own bond with Cinder. When we went on vacation we would always take Cinder with us. The only time we would leave him alone was when we went for our meals (of course, we always returned with food and goodies for him).

Then, without warning, Cinder got sick. He was very lethargic and had no appetite so we brought him to the vet immediately. He hated the vet but we had no choice. It turned out that Cinder had a very bad ear infection and had to stay in the hospital for a week. This was extremely trying on us. The whole family would visit each day to reassure him of our love and let him know that we had not deserted him. Our children were extremely upset because they thought he might die. This was not a fatal illness but we were frightened that Cinder might become deaf.

When we got the test results we found out that Cinder needed surgery and that he had to spend another week in the hospital. The cost of his care was not an issue; we just wanted Cinder better and to come back home to us. So that we could be at the hospital during the surgery, my husband took off from work and the children didn't go to school. After two hours we were told that Cinder would be okay, that she wouldn't be deaf and could come home the next day. You never saw such a happy family; we were jumping and crying at the same time. The children put "Welcome Home" signs all over the house for Cinder. We made sure his favorite blanket was clean and that we had all the proper medications ready. We gave him the best of care and he recovered beautifully.

Cinder was not just a pet to us, he was a full member of our family. He loved the attention we gave him and we loved giving it. To this day I believe he could read or at least understand the "Welcome Home" signs. No one can make me think that he did not understand how much we loved him.

Now we come to the sad part of this story. My oldest daughter, who was seven at the time, was about to make her first Communion. Everyone was excited and we were busy planning a big party. In the afternoon, while we were all running around, Cinder managed to get out of the house. To this day we still don't know how he got away without our knowledge. We were frantic when we found out.

My husband heard what happened and came home from work early. We looked everywhere in the neighborhood and asked everyone if they saw Cinder, but no one had. We didn't know where else to look or what else to do. None of us slept a minute that night.

The next morning a neighbor came to our house to tell us that Cinder had been run over by a car. We ran to the next block where Cinder had been spotted, but when we got there he was already dead. I picked him up, brought him to my bosom and cried like a baby. Everyone was hysterical but the only thing we could do was bring him home until we could make arrangements for his burial. It had to be one of the hardest moments in our lives. To think we would never share his love or be able to give him ours again was unbearable.

We had to go to church for the Communion ceremonies. My daughter was first in line and my husband and I were sitting next to her. We were all crying. The priest came over to me and said, "I know this is an emotional day for you, but you are crying too much." I told him, "It's not my daughter I am crying over, it's the loss of my baby, Cinder." He couldn't quite understand. "What baby?" he asked. I explained that it was the dog I had for eleven years — my "other child." He paused for a moment and told the entire congregation to say a prayer for Cinder. Well, you can imagine my surprise! I was so happy that I began crying again. I thanked him and he kissed me.

After the ceremony some of our friends came over to us and said they were sorry to hear we lost Cinder. Other "friends" thought it was ridiculous that the priest had said what he did. I told them, "I don't care what you think." At that moment, they could all go to hell as far as I was concerned.

I realize now that these people simply did

not appreciate animals. I'm convinced that you must live with and love animals before you can feel the pain of losing them. There is a saying that I believe in wholeheartedly: A person who doesn't love animals cannot love children.

We buried Cinder at Bide-A-Wee pet cemetery on Long Island in a wooden casket with a blue and white lining. Even though we all miss Cinder so much and will never get over losing him, being able to visit him at his grave has been a comfort to us and has strengthened our love as a family.

I want to thank you for letting me share my story with you and the people who will read your book. I hope it will help other people realize that it is normal to feel intense sadness over the death of a pet.

Sincerely,

M.S.M., New York

Little Persons

Dear Kymberly,

I know that I will cry many tears as I write this letter, but perhaps it will help me release some of the terrible sorrow that has consumed me ever since I lost *both* my dog and my cat at almost the same time last year.

Sixteen years ago I brought home a 10-week-old white West Highland terrier puppy who I named Frosty. I became so involved with this puppy and spent just about every waking moment with her. The result of this was that we both learned how to communicate with each other. Frosty was very smart and learned quickly. Before long, she was able to understand everything I said to her.

Frosty loved to play, even up until the last week of her life. Every Christmas we would buy her toys and leave them wrapped beneath the Christmas tree. On Christmas morning, I would say "Go get your presents!" and Frosty would run across the room and rip the paper from the presents. She was a delight to watch — so intelligent, so energetic.

When Frosty was three years old, I got

Chewy, a Blue Persian cat. She was not healthy when we brought her home but after two years of trips to the vet and much caring on my part, she finally became healthy.

Frosty and Chewy were the best of friends; where one went, the other followed. Every morning while my husband and I drank our coffee, we would watch them play with their toys. When my husband came home from work, he would ask Frosty for his slippers and she would find them and then bring them to him. When it was time for bed, I would say "Night, night time," and she would know just what to do. She would run outside then come back in and settle into her bed. Chewy, on the other hand, would head straight for the bedroom, where she slept with her paws wrapped around my neck. For 16 years, this was our routine. Our pets were an integral part of our daily lives.

Even though I never had any children, I never felt lonely or that I was missing out because I had Frosty and Chewy — they were my kids. We were a family and they were with me constantly — when I worked, when I bathed, when I was sick. But this happy family would not last forever...

Not too long ago, Frosty became sick. We discovered that her kidneys were not functioning properly. She was placed on a special diet and had to have her urine analyzed monthly in order to monitor her condition. Around the same time, Chewy developed a cancerous tumor on her paw. We had it removed and prayed that all of the cancerous cells had gone with it. I spent many hours holding, rocking and singing lullabies to the two of them, hoping and praying for their recovery — a recovery that, tragically, was never to occur.

By the end of the year, Frosty's condition

had worsened. She had trouble keeping food down and the test results from the vet revealed that her kidneys had almost stopped functioning. We tried everything, but she was starting to dehydrate and in my heart I knew that she was not going to recover from this. The vet told us that we could give Frosty a few extra days by leaving her in the hospital and putting her on dialysis. She also let us know that the procedure would be a painful one. I didn't want my baby to suffer. I couldn't bear to have Frosty experience any more pain, so we decided to have her put to sleep.

Later that day, I sat in a room at the vet's, holding Frosty in her afghan and talking to her while I stroked her head. The vet came in and asked if I was ready. We put her on a table and I continued talking to her until I knew she was gone. Then I picked her up, wrapped her once again in her afghan and brought her home. I'd never had to do anything like that before and the pain of the whole experience was more than I can describe.

On the evening of Frosty's burial, Chewy started to have problems breathing. I did everything I could think of, but when her breathing didn't improve, I knew it was time to seek professional help. My vet had gone out of town, but I finally located an animal hospital that was open 24 hours a day. While I was doing this, though, Chewy stopped breathing. I performed mouth-to-mouth resuscitation and was able to revive her. As my husband drove us to the hospital, I held Chewy in my arms.

At the hospital, they examined Chewy and placed her in an oxygen cage in an effort to stabilize her. Then they told me that I would have to leave, as that was the hospital's policy. I started crying and told them that not only was Chewy sick, but I had also just lost my dog. But they insisted and reluctantly I left my poor cat. It was five in the morning by the time we got home.

When I arrived the next morning, an attendant was holding an oxygen mask to her face. They told me that Chewy's condition had worsened and that they had found cancer in her lungs. She was not going to get better. Suddenly I was forced to make the same decision for Chewy as I had made for Frosty just the day before. I just couldn't let her suffer any more. I talked and talked to her, hoping that it would calm her so she could lie still and not gasp so much for air. I watched as they gave her the final shot. Her body went limp. Again, I had to watch the agonizing reality of death. The attendant brought me into another room so I could be alone with Chewy's body. I tried to compose myself.

Later that day we buried Chewy next to Frosty. I wanted to die myself. I couldn't believe what had happened. I kept asking myself, "Was it meant to be?" Frosty and Chewy had always been together in life; had God deliberately taken them away at the same time so they could continue to be together? I know that no one lives forever, but it didn't seem possible that both of them could die at the same time.

The pain was so intense. The house seemed so empty. No playtime. No cuddling. I cried and cried. I didn't sleep for weeks. I kept thinking about the last few seconds at the end and it haunted me. It still does. I kept waking up in the middle of the night, imagining I heard one of them crying for me.

I didn't talk much for a few weeks. When someone called or came to the house and asked,

"Where are the troops?" I'd break down. I wasn't hungry and I didn't eat much. I lost weight.

Everyone respected my wishes to be left alone. My husband suffered also. We both cried ourselves to sleep and talked about the babies a lot. Everyone in my family called and tried to console me. My mom was very shaken; she had always brought the babies presents and goodies when she came to visit. I also received a few sympathy cards from friends and one from my vet.

It's been eight months since they've gone and I still cry about it. I miss them so much. I'm not whole without my little family. I can look out my living room window and see their graves at the corner of the yard under a big pine tree, with their own bowl on the top of each grave.

I know I'm not the only person to lose a beloved pet, but that doesn't really make me feel any better. I also know that some people regard pets as less important than people, but not to me. For us, Frosty and Chewy were a large part of our lives. I went through our photo albums and slides and realized that most of the pictures are of Frosty and Chewy. We knew their ways and little quirks and they knew ours; we communicated with each other. Frosty and Chewy were like little persons to us. There was equality between us and a bond of love that nothing could break — not even death, a bond that could not have been stronger had they been human.

Thanks for listening.

Sincerely,

L.D., Massachusetts

The Special Ones

Dear Kymberly,

When people speak of a soulmate, they usually have a very special person in mind. But my soulmate was Sava, my dog. I doubt she even knew that she was a dog, much less a Doberman pinscher, yet somehow we formed a bond that far exceeded most human relationships. Originally, I wasn't planning on keeping the nine-week-old puppy. I had promised a friend that I would find her a home, and within two weeks, I had — inside my heart.

    I've had other pets during my life and I loved them all, but none of them was as special as Sava. At times I swear she could read my mind. I could feel the love flowing between us when our eyes met, when we would be lying face to face at night, breathing each other's breath, or when she lay her head on my chest. My heart would just fill up with my love for her. As the years went by we grew closer and closer. She went everywhere with me.

    One night, nine years later, Sava woke me up with her whimpering. She was lying by my side and she couldn't move, she couldn't even lift her head. I rushed her to the local veterinary school and discovered that she had ruptured a disc in her neck. I scheduled her for surgery even though I was told that the prognosis for this type of injury is not good. Still, I had to do whatever I could for my baby.

Thankfully, after the surgery, Sava was no longer in pain. After months of physical therapy, she wasn't paralyzed any longer, but the damage done to her spinal cord meant that she could never walk again. We had a contraption built to help her get around, but it was still hard for her to walk with it, so I ended up carrying her everywhere she went.

I never gave up hope for Sava's recovery and for the next four years I did everything I could to make life as comfortable as possible. I hired a dog sitter who would stay with her while I was working. Each day he would exercise her legs and massage her neck and shoulders.

All of this was hard work and it was sad for me to see Sava in pain. Sometimes I felt like it was me and Sava against the world. Many people thought I should put her out of her misery, but when I looked into her eyes I didn't see misery — I saw love shining back at me.

But then other things started going wrong. Sava's kidneys started failing and there was evidence that another disc in her neck was pressing on the spinal cord.

One night, four years after her first surgery, I looked in Sava's eyes and I saw pain and I knew it was time. I made arrangements for my vet, God bless him, to come to the house and as I held Sava in my arms, he performed the euthanasia.

I knew putting Sava to sleep was going to be difficult but I wasn't prepared for the pain I felt after she was gone. I felt as if my heart had been torn out of my chest. Because Sava was old and had poor circulation, the anesthetic took longer to work. It is not abnormal, or so I was told, for dogs of Sava's age to cry out, although not in reaction to pain. When Sava cried out I thought I too was going to die. Not only did I feel terrible about losing her but I also began to feel guilty about having her put down. It seemed as though I had lost my best friend and my child at the same time. I was really not sure that I could survive.

For the most part, my family and friends were supportive of me. They were well aware of the special bond Sava and I shared. People sent me sympathy cards and made donations to humane societies in Sava's memory. A dear friend did a charcoal drawing of Sava that I framed and hung over my bed.

It has now been over a year since I lost my Sava, but thanks to a pet support group that was started by a caring person who, like me, had lost a beloved animal friend, things have been a little easier. It helps to share the stories of our dear ones and to know that others have loved their babies almost as much as I loved Sava.

Still, there are times when I am overcome with the loss almost as if it had happened just yesterday. I still miss her so very much and I know my life will never be the same without her. But I also believe that we will be together again in Heaven, so I can bear our separation for the time being.

Once in a while, I am even able to smile when I think of how her ears turned out to the sides like little bat wings or how she'd back up to sit in a chair like a person would or lie down and cross her front legs like a lady.

    I hope our story will be of some help to you. It would be an honor to Sava's memory if you include my letter in your book. Thank you for taking the time and effort to try to ease the suffering of those of us who have lost special friends.

For Sava

They come into our lives,
These special ones,
For much too short a time.
And even though we are blessed
with the precious love they bring,
We will never again be the same.
For once your heart belongs to an angel,
The rest of the world seems to lose its magic
when they go away.
Almost as if a part of your soul, too,
has gone with them.

Sincerely,

P.T., Michigan

We Had a Bond

Dear Kymberly,

When I heard about the book you were writing, I knew that I had to send you my story about what I went through when my cat, Magnum, died. I don't want anyone to have to suffer like I did, so I hope my story will help someone in some way. I also have another reason for writing to you: not only do I love to talk about my cat, but I *need* to tell someone about what happened.

After more than 13 years of working at the hospital, I was laid off. Feeling down about being unemployed and having a lot of time on my hands, I thought getting a kitten might help me forget all my problems. I also wanted to get a boy kitten because even though I had a daughter whom I love dearly, I always wanted a boy. Because I couldn't have any more children, I thought a boy kitten could be the son I never had.

Magnum was a six-week-old kitten when we got him. My husband said he was ugly, but I thought he was the most precious thing I had ever seen. With so much time on my hands, I petted and pampered him and played with him all day. It didn't take long for me to fall in love with him.

Magnum was such a sweet cat and I want to tell you just a few of the things he did that made him so special and made me love him so much. His first and favorite toy was a red rabbit's foot. Over the years he had rabbit's feet in all colors, but he loved his red one, which I still have. I would throw it and say, "Ready, set, go!" and he would go get it. Soon I had him fetching like a dog. As he got bigger, he became smarter and smarter and I loved him more and more. There was a bond between us, an understanding that no one else in the family had.

On Magnum's first Christmas I bought some toys for his stocking. He was watching when I hid the presents in the kitchen cabinet until later when I could wrap them. I guess he just couldn't wait until Christmas because the next day I found him up on the washing machine, stretching as far as he could to open the cabinet and get his toys out. He knew they were for him!

A couple of years later, Honeybunny, a gray striped cat with white paws, came into our lives. When my daughter found her under our tree, she was soaking wet and expecting kittens. We brought her into our home and cleaned her up. It didn't take long for all of us to fall in love with her. She filled our lives with joy and Magnum soon grew to love her too. They were like brother and sister.

Magnum loved it when I held him in my arms and rocked him like a baby. He would use the potty whenever I told him to and at night all I had to say to him was "Night night time" and he would get on his favorite blanket and go to sleep. In the middle of the night he would come to my bed and rub his nose on my face and then lay in my arms.

    When I got a new job and wasn't home all day, I missed Magnum terribly. But when I came home, he was always waiting at the door to greet me. He always brought me so much joy.

    This next part is very hard for me to write. I am already crying so hard just thinking about it that I can hardly see the paper, but I need to tell you what happened. When Magnum was four, he started to have trouble with his kidneys. It got so bad that he could hardly urinate. I took him to the vet and he tried different medicines but nothing helped. I was so upset that Magnum was sick that I couldn't sleep and I cried all the time because he wasn't getting any better. My husband thought that we should put Magnum out of his misery and he would constantly pressure me about this. The doctor said that he had done all he could. His suggestion to me was to put my cat in a rabbit cage and keep him outside. That way I wouldn't have to deal with the mess that resulted from his incontinence. I would have rather died.

    Magnum got worse and so did my nerves; the doctor bills, lack of sleep and the pressure from my husband to have him put to sleep were tearing me apart. Of course the worst thing was that my poor cat was sick and hurting. I was so torn up, I thought I was going to have a nervous breakdown. Magnum meant the world to me, but I knew that soon I was going to have to make a decision that I really didn't want to make. I didn't sleep at all that night and while I was at work the next day I just sat there and cried. Finally I picked up the phone and called the vet and told him I wanted to have Magnum put to sleep.

    I went home and rocked Magnum in my arms

for about an hour before leaving for the vet. When we got there, the nurse put us in this little room. I thought that my heart would break in two when Magnum climbed up on my lap and put both his little paws around my neck. I wept all over him, begging him to just use his potty so we could go home and resume our happy life together. For four years he had always been good and always did what I said and now he was so sick and I felt like I was letting him down.

    I had no more money for further medical tests (even though I don't know that anything could have helped at that point) and I felt that putting him to sleep was my only choice. What a choice — to kill someone that I loved as much as life itself.

    When the nurse walked away with Magnum, I felt like someone had taken a giant knife and ripped my heart out of my chest. As soon as the nurse left with Magnum, I suddenly started to panic — I couldn't go through with this! — and I ran after them...but it was too late. That quickly Magnum was gone. We wrapped him in his favorite blanket and I took him with me. I was so sick over what happened that I threw up. A part of me died that day and I have never gotten over it.

    I took Magnum home and rocked him for hours. My head hurt so much that I went to bed and laid him beside me. We stayed there until my husband came home. He didn't know that I had gone through with the euthanasia and when he saw Magnum lying there next to me, he thought he was sleeping. I was hysterical as I told him that I had killed my baby. He took Magnum outside and buried him in the back yard. I followed and sat at the grave for hours. I was so sick with grief that I couldn't eat.

The following days and months were rough for me. I would cry myself to sleep every night holding Magnum's picture to my chest. After six weeks of doing this, I thought that maybe I would stop thinking about him so much if I put his picture away. But it didn't help...nothing did. I just couldn't get him out of my mind.

Magnum used to make a swishing sound when he walked and for about a year after he was gone I would actually think I could hear him walking across the floor. I wanted to talk to other people about him so much because I felt that if I talked about him, maybe somehow it would bring him back. But no one in my family wanted to hear about it. I was even asked not to mention his name in the house any more! Mom wouldn't listen — she said I was crazy for crying over a cat. My sisters didn't like animals and they didn't understand what I was going through. I even resorted to asking God to raise him from the dead. I cried day and night. I cried the whole time I was in church. Everybody there thought I had lost my mind because I wouldn't tell them what was wrong. I knew that I needed some kind of help because I just couldn't go on like that. So I called several veterinarians to see if they knew of any support groups I could go to. They gave me the name of one, but it was too far away.

I couldn't find any help, so I kept the pain inside and cried to myself when no one was around. I wouldn't just cry, I would go into hysterics and hit the wall and scream, "God, why did he have to die?" I tried blaming God and then my husband but I knew all along that it had been *my* decision to put Magnum to sleep. I hated myself for what I had done.

    When I begged my husband to dig Magnum up so I could hold him one more time, he told me that I needed to get help. I am a Christian so I asked God to help me get through the grief. I decided to put my energy into caring for my other cat, Honeybunny. She missed Magnum too and would go through the house looking for him. For three days after Magnum died, she wouldn't eat. It wasn't fair for me to ignore her because I was so consumed with grief for Magnum. This was a very good decision and it helped a lot even though, of course, it didn't make my terrible pain over losing Magnum go away. I was able to love her and she felt it and loved me back.

    But my troubles were not over. Two years later Honeybunny began to get sick. I couldn't bring myself to take her to the vet because it brought back too many memories of Magnum, so my daughter had to do it. This time my husband stepped in and when Honeybunny started to bleed internally, he made the decision that she had to be put to sleep.

    I was still grieving over Magnum and now my Honeybunny was taken away too. Life just seemed so unfair. It's been four years now since Magnum's death and two since Honeybunny's. Things are a little better, but I will never really get over losing these animals that I loved so much. I still cry when I get their pictures out.

    I have four other cats now, but I learned a painful lesson with Magnum and Honeybunny. I will never allow myself to love these cats as I did my first two. It seems like everything I really love goes away. The four cats I have now are precious, but I never want to experience the hurt of loss again.

Maybe loss is inevitable when you love someone or something deeply, but knowing this doesn't make anything easier. I pray to God that no one has to feel the kind of hurt that I have.

Good luck and God bless you for caring,

L.B., North Carolina

The Caregiver

Dear Kymberly,

Five months ago, we lost our dog, Fuzzy. She was 15 years and 23 days old and we had her for every minute of that time. A bona fide member of our family, she saw our children grow up and she saw our grandchildren become part of our family. She was loved.
    Fuzzy was born in a corner on our back porch, arriving just as my youngest son got home from school. Of the seven puppies, Fuzzy was the only long-haired female and we decided to keep her. She carried the collie markings perfectly, from the ruff to the white stockings.
    Fuzzy was stubborn and had a mind of her own. She trained us all well as her mother had trained her. She had the collie streak of perfection: never sit around with muddy fur and always look your best. But she had the hound playfulness: "Nevertheless, I like to dig in the dirt and play in the water!" She hated to chase balls. She would go get a ball once just to show us she knew what we wanted and then she would hide it and go do what she wanted to do. She did the same thing with the

mail. She would get it to show her superior intelligence and then she would drop it in the dirt so no one would ever ask her to get it again.

Fuzzy's one calling in life was to take care of her family. She was a canine Florence Nightingale. If one of us was sick in bed, or, heaven help us, coughing, she'd get right on the job by crawling in bed with the patient. She never left their side for a minute. If someone coughed, she was right there trying to look down their throat. We are talking about a 50-pound dog here — and you haven't been nursed until you've been nursed by a 50-pound dog.

She loved to go hiking, but drove herself and the rest of us crazy trying to herd us into a line so that she could watch all at once. Sometimes, if the hill was steep, she would let me hold onto her so I wouldn't fall, especially going down. She would even pull as we went uphill. I trusted her and her feet never slipped; as long as I held onto her, I knew I was safe.

The only time I can remember Fuzzy getting in trouble (except for eating an occasional potted plant when she was a puppy) involved a beautiful cake that I had made for Thanksgiving. I set it on our bed until we were ready to go to my sister-in-law's house and when I wasn't looking, she ate it. I was so angry! I looked at her and the ruined cake that I had put so much work into and I scolded her severely. I was so mad I took some of the remaining cake and stuffed it in her mouth. I told her if she liked cake so much, she may as well eat it all. She spat it out disdainfully and she never again took food off the bed (I also never again left food on the bed). She was sorry and every time anyone even said the word cake from then on, she hung her head.

We had many adventures during her lifetime. The kids grew up and graduated from high school and college and then got married. Soon grandchildren began arriving and as much as she had loved our children, Fuzzy did not seem to like the grandchildren. They were always touching her and she treated them like "dirty little creatures" (she may have learned this from her mother who thought little children were dirty and who hated anything dirty or sticky). However, a perfect dog never harms even dirty little creatures, so she would only growl at them. She didn't use a menacing or frightening growl, just a "Fuzzy growl." She would growl when they simply looked at her. I would ask them, "What did you do to Fuzzy to make her growl?" It took me awhile to catch on that she was trying to get them in trouble. I swear that she would smile when they got scolded for bothering her.

Yet Fuzzy must have loved my grandchildren after all because her greatest act of heroism concerned the oldest one who was four at the time. My husband and I and my grandchild were walking with Fuzzy when suddenly a large German shepherd came running at us with his teeth bared, ready to attack. He was running right at my grandchild when Fuzzy jumped between them. They fought (the German shepherd bit off half of Fuzzy's ear) and then it was over. If Fuzzy had not jumped between them, my grandchild would have been badly bitten. Fuzzy may have lost part of her ear, but you have to make some sacrifices to be a heroine.

In 1987 Fuzzy developed arthritis in her back legs and we also realized that her hearing wasn't as good as it used to be. The vet who examined her said she was healthy otherwise, but Fuzzy took a different view. I think she decided she was going to die. She lay around without moving and she didn't want to do anything. We'd call her and she would just look at us. I also thought that she was going to die and I even considered putting her to sleep but I couldn't go through with it. She wasn't in pain; she just didn't want to go on.

In November of that year, my daughter gave us a new puppy. My husband was completely against the idea. But then a strange thing happened. Fuzzy was suddenly back to her old self. She could get around just fine and she could even hear things again. She decided that she had to take care of that puppy and she did. She had a new purpose in life and it gave her a reason to live.

Fuzzy became a new mother and the puppy became the child that Fuzzy had apparently always wanted. Fuzzy taught her all the tricks — how to open the door with your nose; how to scratch on the door when you want to come in; how to get your bowl and bring it in the kitchen when you are hungry; how to ignore people when you don't want to do something; how to get on the bed and find just the right spot when no one is home; how to lie in the sun on a cold day. Needless to say, we kept the puppy. I couldn't believe the "new" Fuzzy. It was incredible that she decided to keep on living so that she could mother the newest member of our family.

Cinnamon grew into a fine dog. Even though Fuzzy's arthritis continued to get worse, she still followed us from room to room, she still growled at the grandchildren and took care of her adopted child. By April she was in a bad way; she would go off by herself and lie down behind the bed where no one would bother her. She no longer growled at the kids and that was a clear sign that we were close to the end.

The vet said I would know when it was time. I did whatever I could to take care of her: I hand-fed her, I petted her and loved her more than ever. Then on a Sunday, I discovered that Fuzzy could hardly move. On Monday morning she couldn't move at all. She couldn't even get up to do her business and she so hated to be dirty. In desperation I called the vet, but when I tried to speak to him, I was so upset I couldn't make a sound. When my husband called to see how Fuzzy was, I was crying so hard I couldn't talk to him. He had to call and make the arrangements with the vet to have Fuzzy euthanized.

When my husband got home, we put Fuzzy in a box and took her to the vet's. I was crying so hard I couldn't see straight. Soon the doctor came out of his examination room and told us it was over. He put Fuzzy in a new box and we brought her home and buried her by the apple trees in the yard. The vet told us that Fuzzy was a special dog and that we must be a special family to have taken such good care of her for so long.

We will always remember Fuzzy. She liked to eat watermelon right off the rind, but she wouldn't eat a pickle for love or money. She would tell us when the phone was ringing and she knew when it was time for her heartworm pill every night. She knew she wasn't allowed on the bed, but she slept there anyway.

Fuzzy had the most beautiful, soft, silky fur. I cut some off just before we took her in that last day and put it in a plastic bag. Now when I touch it, all of her beauty and specialness come back to me. Fuzzy was there when I had pneumonia and she was there for me when the kids left home. She was there to growl at the first grandchild and the second, third, fourth and fifth. She was there to run and play with the children. She loved tug-of-war and swimming in the ditch. She hated to have wet feet and always made a point to stay on the porch till they dried. She was a stubborn, lovable 50 pounds of friendship and loyalty and we miss her terribly.

It did me a world of good to write this letter to you. It is important for people to know that when a loved pet dies, they need to remember all the good times they had with their pet and all the things they learned. Dogs are great teachers. In reality, people don't take care of their dogs, their dogs take care of them.

Sincerely,

R.C., California

Not "Only a Dog"

Dear Kymberly,

I lost Kachina my golden retriever last year. About a year before she died, I found out that she had cancer — an advanced case of melanoma. After she had surgery, the doctor told me he was pretty sure that he had removed all of the cancerous tissue that was in her mouth and throat. He must have had his doubts though, because he told me to go see a colleague of his who specialized in oral cancer. Two weeks later I brought Kachina to the second veterinarian and, sure enough, he discovered more cancer and I had to leave Kachina with him for a second round of surgery. This time the cancer was further down her throat and part of her left jaw had to be removed.

Because pets were not allowed in my apartment building, Kachina had to stay with my parents who lived about five miles from me. After her operation, I went to their house every day to be with my dog. Soon I noticed that Kachina wasn't doing so well and when I brought her back to the vet, he said that the cancer had spread and that he would have to remove the rest of the left side of her jaw.

    After that, Kachina could only eat baby food or dog food that I would purée in a blender and then feed to her. Because the left side of her jaw was now gone, her tongue always hung out of her mouth. But she was still so beautiful to me. I did everything I could to care for her and make her happy. I would take her to the park and buy her yogurt and ice cream. When she was done eating, I had to wipe her face like she was a child.

    Kachina was 10 years old when all this happened — a good lifespan for a golden retriever, or so I was told. I was also told that her disease was incurable and that there was no way to know when the cancer would end her life.

    I could not stand the thought of losing her, so I decided to "solve" the problem by ending my own life. I figured that if I died before she did, I wouldn't be there to suffer the pain of losing her. Now, looking back, I'm glad that I didn't go ahead with my plan because by staying alive, I was able to take care of my sick dog and make the rest of her life as happy as I could.

    By the time I took Kachina in for her next check-up, she really wasn't doing well. She had lost a lot of weight and she didn't want to be around anyone. Maybe she began losing her will to go on living. Even though I knew that we were going to have to put her to sleep, I didn't want to think about it. Being responsible for ending the life of my closest companion was too horrible. The vet gave me a choice: either I could bring her back in two weeks for another examination or he could put her to sleep right then and there. The whole thing seemed so unfair. Why did it have to be my decision? I didn't know what to do. I wish I knew if she was in pain. Did she want to die? If only Kachina could have told me what she wanted.

    I decided that I had no choice but to have her put to sleep that day. I watched as the vet inserted an IV and administered the fatal drug. Kachina was lying on a woolly blanket and I lay down next to her. The vet told me to keep talking to her as she slowly went to sleep, but I found that I couldn't say much. All I could do was cry and put my face in her fur and tell her how much I loved her. As difficult as it was for me, it did seem like a very peaceful way to die.

    That was 11 months ago. Not a day has gone by that I don't think of Kachina. I had her cremated and I buried the urn in my parents' back yard. There's a stone on her grave and my brother planted my favorite flowers all around it. Every time I visit my parents, I lay fresh flowers beside the stone.

    My friends and acquaintances were not very understanding when I told them about Kachina's death and how sad I was. They "allowed" me to feel bad for about three days and then they lost their patience with me. "She was only a dog, so get over it," some of them told me. Maybe to them Kachina was "only a dog," but to me, a single adult without any children, Kachina was everything — my family and my best friend. Still people found it inconceivable that I could be so upset over the loss of a dog. They must not have had any understanding of the kind of relationship that can develop between a person and an animal companion. To them, a dog does not deserve the kind of grief that I was displaying. They thought it was strange that I was upset for more than a few days. What would they think if they knew that I'll be upset until the day comes when I am with Kachina again? I finally made the decision not to talk to people about Kachina anymore; I've realized that I can't make them understand my grief and the depth of my love for her.

    I still agonize over my decision to have Kachina put to sleep. I don't know if I did the right thing and in a way I feel as if I killed her. Maybe if I had taken her home with me that day she would have lived longer than anyone thought. After all, she had already lived five months beyond what the doctors had predicted, so maybe she would have been okay. I can only hope that if Kachina was in pain, maybe I helped her. Maybe I proved my love for her. Maybe she understood what I was trying to do. I guess there are a lot of maybes.

    I'm not ready to get another dog and I'm not sure if I ever will be. In looking back over everything that happened, I've come to the conclusion that the good times I had with Kachina were well worth the hurt I feel now. I just hope they were worth it for Kachina, too.

Sincerely,

E.M.A., California

When Part of Me Died

Dear Kymberly,

I meant to write to you sooner, but I've found that writing about my loss brings up all the pain again and I've had a hard time finding the courage. Even though it is hard, it is important for me to share my story.

I wanted a dog ever since I was five years old. My mother was afraid of dogs and wouldn't let me have one, but I thought of nothing else and longed for the wonderful day when I could finally have a puppy and best friend. It wasn't until my senior year in college, when I was preparing to go to law school, that I decided it was now or never. I looked through the paper, found a breeder and went to see her Sheltie puppies. From the moment I saw Sadie there was no doubt that she was the one for me. The runt of the litter, she was a beautiful tricolor, full of fun and energy. When we would go for walks, people would stop their cars to get a better look and pet her. Everyone who met her came away amazed.

Sadie and I developed a psychic connection. She understood almost everything I said and even when she wasn't with me, I could feel her presence. Despite her lifelong uneasiness with dogs, my mother fell in love with Sadie and actually slept with her when I came for visits. I was living in California at the time, on a beautiful, spacious property — all wooded and peaceful and quiet. Sadie loved to spend her days outside, lying in the grass and watching the world go by. She was never one to stray, and on our walks I rarely had to use a leash. She stayed right by me and always came immediately when I called.

One early autumn morning, I let her outside as I always did while I got her kibble ready. My roommate had a dog who was high-strung and not very smart when it came to cars. He was always running into the street and rushing up and down the block. Sadie never joined him. On this morning, at the precise moment I let her out, a delivery truck was coming up the road. Trucks were the one thing she hated with a passion, and even if she saw one through a window, the sight of it would agitate her.

The two dogs ran outside and I heard them barking. I was two steps from the door, just about to call her, when a heard a high, squeaky yelp. Dressed only in pajamas, I ran outside to see the love of my life lying in the road with the other dog standing over her. When I got to her, Sadie was shaking and quivering. The worst nightmare of my life was unfolding before me, and I couldn't think of what to do. I kept calling to her, and then I saw the truck's driver lean out the side window. "You hit my dog!" I shouted at her. Her only response was, "She got in my way." She then drove away, leaving me alone in the road with my poor dog. When I think back on it now, I usually envision myself grabbing or shaking the driver, trying to make her realize what a precious life she had taken by driving too fast and not paying attention.

    I scooped Sadie up, ran in the house and called 911. The operator refused to help me; she told me to go to a vet and then hung up. There was no one around and I knew I had to act immediately. I couldn't tell if she was breathing, but I convinced myself that she was in a coma; she looked okay to me and there were no signs of bleeding.

    I threw on some clothes, took Sadie in my arms and ran out of the house with only my car keys — no money, no ID, all the doors wide open. I got in the car, laid Sadie on the seat next to me and took off as fast as I could. I was too upset to have been driving, but I needed someone to help Sadie immediately. The speed limit in the canyon was 45 mph, but I must have been going 75. I took a turn too fast and smashed into the side of a cliff. My car ricocheted and went straight for the guard rail. This is it, I thought to myself as my front tire went over the top. I thought of my parents and how awful it would be for them to find both of us dead at the bottom of the canyon, never knowing how such a thing could happen.

    I heard a loud bang and the car shook. My head hit something, my glasses flew off and the car stopped. Without a moment's thought, I grabbed my glasses, took Sadie in my arms, pushed the mangled door open and ran out into the middle of the road, yelling to the people who had stopped to please, *please* help me. One of them offered to drive me to the vet in town. The whole time I begged him to please hurry. I just kept looking into Sadie's eyes, asking her if she could hear me and telling her to hold on. She felt warm and her nose was wet, so I clung to the belief that there was still hope. I tried to will her to live; I tried to burn it into her with my eyes. I had been through some very rough times since I moved to California, and she was all I had in the world. God would never be so cruel as to take her away from me after everything I'd been through.

When we finally got to the vet, I ran inside and yelled, "Please help me! My dog has been hit by a car!" The receptionist grabbed Sadie and ran in the back while I paced, wringing my hands, praying hysterically and looking pretty wild. Finally the vet came in, looked at me with a stony face and said, "She's dead." I sort of collapsed and then I begged, "Please don't say that. Please, isn't there anything you can do? She is my whole life!" The vet looked up from her clipboard and snapped, "What do you want from me? She was dead when you brought her in here." She then turned on her heel and walked out. No one who worked in that clinic offered me a kind word or any sort of comfort. The receptionist did say that I could go back and see Sadie and take as long as I needed to get myself together, but that was the only comforting I received. While I was in the room with Sadie, I heard the vet ask, "Is she *still* in there? How long is she going to take?"

I had always been so particular in choosing wonderful, caring vets, but my regular doctor was too far away to help me in this emergency. How awful it made me feel that the only vet I could find was this horrible woman who, I found out later, had several complaints lodged against her because of her ineptness and uncaring attitude.

The day just went from one horrible incident to the next. I called my family — the hardest call I ever made — to tell them the tragic news. Living in another state, they felt so helpless to do anything for me, and their hearts ached with grief. Then called a friend and she took the day off from work to drive me to the pet cemetery where Sadie was to be cremated. One of the most painful things I ever did in my life was to answer the questions the secretary at the cemetery had to ask me, write her a check and then hand my Sadie over to her to take away. Never to sleep with her again, never to hear her bark or see her "happy dance" or smell her fur, never to hold her again or have her at my side. The pain was numbing. I decided to bury Sadie's ashes in my parents' backyard where she had spent so many happy hours, and where I knew I would always be able to visit.

    The word got out and I received phone calls and cards and letters from friends all over the country . I never got any sort of negative response from my friends, because they all knew how inseparable Sadie and I were. Many of them cried and said that they'd never met a dog like Sadie.

    For the next several weeks I saw the world through a veil of tears. It was the beginning of a very bad period for me — perhaps the lowest I've ever been. Nothing mattered to me, I quit my job, got involved with the wrong men, made bad decisions and pondered suicide. Nothing would relieve the overwhelming pain of losing Sadie.

    I flew home to stay with my folks for a couple weeks to bury Sadie and visit her breeder. The breeder knew that I had lost Sadie and suggested that I might like to come over and see a new litter of puppies. While I knew that no other dog could replace Sadie, I found that just being around the puppies lightened my heart a little. I ended up choosing two: a tricolor just like Sadie that I named Kady, and a blue merle that I named Callie. I couldn't take them with me right away as they were only three weeks old, but my breeder promised to bring them with her on an upcoming car trip to California. I will never forget her kindness to me and her special efforts to help me mend my broken heart.

In the three years that have passed since Sadie's death, not a day has gone by that I don't think about her and feel her loss. Nothing will ever fill the empty spot in my heart. I used to send flowers for my parents to place on Sadie's grave on her birthday and the anniversary of her death, but it was made me too sad so I stopped. But my mother still sends me a card on both of those days, reaffirming her love and support.

A couple of times in the beginning I called a pet support hotline that was run out of the local university and they were very kind and helpful. One person I spoke to at length was a student at the veterinary school. After we spoke, she wrote me a four-page letter in which she suggested books I could read and groups I could join to help me with my grief and she also gave me the names of local therapists who specialized in pet loss and bereavement. Her comforting words and suggestions meant a lot to me.

I made a beautiful album of Sadie's life. In it I put this letter, the cards and letters I received after her death and photos of Sadie. From time to time when I really miss her, I take it down and look at it with my dogs, Kady and Callie, but it's still pretty painful for me. But even if I don't look at it, it's a comfort for me to know it's there.

I will always feel guilty about the way Sadie died. She never *ever* ran into the street, even if she was chasing a ball or a squirrel, she would go as far as the curb and then stop. But this road had no curb, and this one time, she just must have forgotten. I've relived the day of her death a million times in my mind and heart, and I cry each time, wishing and wishing that I could make one thing — anything — different to alter the course of that day. But it always plays out the same way, with the same dreadful ending.

Strangely enough, I decided to bring Sadie to work with me on the day before her death. As she and I were playing during my lunch break, one of my employer's children came up to me and asked, "What would you do if Sadie died?" Without hesitation I replied, "I would die too." Part of me did die along with Sadie, but the rest of me is struggling to go on. It does seem silly to some people I guess, but she was really like my own child, and they say losing your child is the most stressful thing you can go through. I believe it.

It has been very difficult for me to put this down on paper, but it has also been therapeutic. I hope it will help other people who are grieving.

Very truly yours,

L.W., California

Beloved Friends

Dear Kymberly,

My letter tells the remarkable story of friendship between my two horses, Pepper and Screwball. Pepper, my quarter horse mare, was black with a white blaze. Screwball was a quarter horse and an Arab cross gelding. A sorrel in color, he came into my life when he was just a year old. When they died, Screwball was 20 and Pepper was 19.

    For more than a decade, the two horses lived peacefully on 14 acres of pasture dotted with big oak trees and a meandering creek. After 11 years, the property was reclaimed by its owner, and my family had to move. I was able to find a three-acre tract of pasture not far away with a barn and an electric fence. For added security I put locks on the gates.

    My last happy memory of my beloved friends, Pepper and Screwball, was the day I went over to the pasture to remove the lock from the gate so that a friend could get some hay from the barn. I remember a long, leisurely visit during which I brushed them and fed them carrots. The next day, I awoke in the very early morning to an insistent pounding at my door. My friends were outside and they were in an excited state. They had come to tell me that Pepper and Screwball had gotten out, even though the gate was latched, and that both horses had been hit by a car. My husband and I rushed to our pickup truck. As we drove along I saw a horse in the ditch along the side of the road. I remember saying to myself, "No, that's not Pepper." When we were closer, I got out and switched on my flashlight. What I saw made me feel that my heart might give out. There was Pepper, my sweet baby girl, her eyes still open but the life gone out of her. As I closed her eyes, I remember telling her how much I loved her and how sorry I was that this was how we had to part company. I hugged her and kissed her goodbye.

    I then thought of Screwball. I had been told that he had been put in a nearby pasture. We drove the pickup into the field, but there was no sign of Screwball. I got out and began looking around. Finally I heard him; he was down in the grass and trying to get up. I checked him over and I knew in my heart that he was soon going to join Pepper. I ran to a neighbor's house and called my vet. When I told him what happened, he promised to come immediately.

    Screwball was still struggling to get up when I returned. I lay down beside him to try to keep him calm, but he kept trying to stand up and it was clear that he was anxious to find Pepper. The vet arrived and after examining Screwball, he sadly shook his head. When I looked into Screwball's eyes, it seemed as if he was pleading with me to let him go. The vet gave him a shot and within two minutes he was gone. It was the best but most horrible choice I have ever had to make.

After giving my family the awful news, my husband and I went to our pasture to look at the gate the horses had escaped through. Someone had unlatched it and left it wide open. To this day I have no idea who could have done such a heartless thing. Later in the day I got a call from the boy who had hit my horses. He told me he was driving only 30 miles an hour and because it was dark, he didn't see the horses until it was too late. He said he was unable to stop in time. He added that he needed $3,000 to pay for the damage to his car. I told him I had no money to give him, and anyway, I didn't think I was liable. The boy called again the next day. This time he said that the damage was more like $4,000. I asked him if Pepper had died instantly and he said it took about half an hour for her to die. I told him not to call again. It struck me that this was the first time in 23 years that I didn't have a horse in my life.

About a month later, the sheriff came to advise me that I was being charged with having "livestock at large." I was shocked to learn that if I was found guilty, I could face a year in jail or a $2,500 fine. I contacted an attorney who advised me to get my friends to write letters on my behalf. I was able to get 15 letters from people who stated that I was a responsible horse owner. The charge was dropped.

Not long afterward, I was served with court papers stating that the driver intended to sue me for half a million dollars in damages. He claimed a wide range of complaints resulting from the accident, from sprains and lacerations to neck and back injuries. The attorney I hired told me that I could countersue for the value of my horses, but I could not collect for pain and suffering even though I lost two wonderful and irreplaceable friends.

I know that Pepper and Screwball are now in a better place and I hope that they are together. Not a day goes by that I am not reminded of them in one way or another. When the time comes that I am ready to have a horse in my life again, I won't get one without also finding a companion. Horses get so lonely when they are alone. Whenever you have animals in your life, you know that sooner or later you will have to deal with their death. I knew that with Pepper and Screwball, if one of them was failing, I might very well have to put both of them down because they could not have lived without each other. This may sound cruel, but it would have been what they wanted — to die as they lived, together.

Thank you for letting me share my story,

T.M., Oregon

My Furry Soulmate

Dear Kymberly,

Although I have lost four geriatric animal friends in the last six months, the first one to die, Chou Chou Pekingese, was the hardest because she was my furry soulmate.

It was late at night and I was home alone when Chou Chou fell through the stairway railing from the second floor to the first and broke her spine. I called a vet who handled emergencies and I rushed her to his office. She was severely injured and in shock. So was I.

The vet took one look at Chou Chou Pekingese and said that there was no hope of recovery. He told me that the best thing to do was to put her down. I was faced with the hardest decision of my life — whether or not to end my darling companion's suffering by ending her life. I knew that I had no other choice — for all the love and joy she had given me, I couldn't let her suffer. Any other decision would have been selfish.

I put my arms around Chou Chou while the vet administered the injection and I looked into her eyes until I knew that she was gone. They wrapped her in a pink flowered blanket and I sat with her until my husband came to get me. I was much too upset to drive home by myself.

My friends and family were kind and loving and I was very lucky to have such a large support system. They seemed to understand that because I didn't have any children, Chou Chou was the closest thing to being my child. They also realized that although I loved my other dog and my two cats, Chou Chou had been my favorite because she had been with me the longest. I received many sympathy cards and felt lucky to have so much support.

Several months later, I heard about a pet grief therapist who held regular meetings for people grieving over the loss of their pets. I attended these meetings for several months and listened to other people talk about the pain of losing their pets. I found it was helpful to hear what others had to say. I also found that because I had such a strong support network of friends and family, my adjustment to the loss of my dog was perhaps less painful than it was for other people.

I had Chou Chou cremated and her ashes put in a Chinese urn. Last year, when I went to China, I took some of her ashes with me. When I was in Peking, I scattered her ashes in a pretty garden within the walls of the Forbidden City. I decided to do this because I felt that, in a way, I was bringing her home to her ancestors. Originally, Pekingese dogs were bred only in the Forbidden City and only the dignitaries who lived there were allowed to even look at them. I felt very honored to have had the love of one of these special dogs.

I was so lucky to have had a strong network of friends and family members to help me during my time of grief. I know that there are many people who have lost a pet who do not have this kind of support. Also, I learned that a pet's death can be more painful than even a relative's death because many people don't think that it's acceptable to mourn openly over the death of a pet. As a result, many people internalize their grief and this can make a terrible situation even worse. If anyone reading this letter falls into this category, I would highly recommend finding a support group where you can be around people who will understand you, who will listen to you and to whom you can express your feelings openly.

I hope my letter will be of help to you.

Sincerely,

M.B.W., Pennsylvania

Tears for Joy, Tears for Sorrow

Dear Kymberly,

When I came to this country in 1979, I had only enough English to do the simplest things. Because I didn't have a driver's license, most of my time was spent in and around the apartment complex where I lived. When my husband started his own business, I was even more alone. He felt sorry for me, I think, so one Christmas he went to the local shelter to get me a cat. Unfortunately, the one he chose was very sick and it only survived a short time. A couple weeks later, a friend took me to look at some kittens. That's when I got Alibaba.

    He was a cute gray tabby, only 12 weeks old. He was very shy and it took a lot of patience to teach him what he needed to know, but I quickly grew to love him with all my heart. Alibaba enjoyed his brushings and seemed to appreciate all the attention I gave to him. We did almost everything together except take a bath.

    When I started working, I got Alibaba a playmate so he would have some company while I was gone. Still, the moment I got home, he wanted only to be with me. He would greet me at the door and follow me all around the house until it was bedtime. I'd say, "Let's go to bed" and that's where he would stay until it was time for his feeding in the morning.

It seemed like Alibaba had almost every illness a cat could get. I spent many nights at the veterinary hospital with him and each time the experience filled me with fear. I did not want to lose him for anything in the world.

Late one autumn, Alibaba had a severe attack of a kind that was new to me and I took him to the vet immediately. After an all-night fight for his life, I took him home. The vet diagnosed hyperthyroid disease and prescribed some pills to be taken twice a day. Alibaba responded very well to them and even started to play again.

One day the following spring, I came home from work and he greeted me lovingly as he always did. I sat down so he could jump up on my lap. As he tried, Alibaba fell backward and lay completely still. I tried everything I could think of to revive him, but nothing would bring him back.

My vet said Alibaba had suffered a severe heart attack and that he died without pain, but the pain I felt in losing him would not go away. After two weeks of crying, I still could not let go of him. I couldn't even imagine life without him.

My husband buried Alibaba behind the house, but after talking to my sister-in-law, I decided that it would be better to move him to a pet cemetery. He was buried in a nice place under a tree that I knew he'd love and I go there as many times as I can. Spending time at his resting place has strengthened me.

There are times when I still can't believe that Alibaba is gone. At first even talking about him was just too painful for me. Though I do not believe that it is possible to transfer love from a departed pet to a living one, I can say that it helps to open your home to a new animal friend. I have two other cats and have just adopted a kitten, but my tears of joy that they are now a part of my life will always contain tears of sorrow for another part that is gone.

C.Y., California

I Am Not Comforted

Dear Kymberly,

When I saw your letter in *I Love Cats* magazine, I had to write to you. You see, my sweet baby died just a few days ago and even if you can't use my letter in your book, it might ease my pain to tell you Snowball's story.

    When I was growing up in Chicago we had a family dog, but ever since I can remember, I always wanted a cat. My mom hates cats and my younger brothers were allergic to them, so I wasn't able to have a cat until I left home. When my family moved to Tucson, I stayed in Chicago to finish nursing school. At the time I was engaged to be married but when things didn't work out, I also moved to Tucson. The adjustment was hard and I was sad and depressed. I felt that I had made a mistake by moving.

    Then near Christmas, around ten years ago, my brother gave me a gift that changed my life. He had a secret smile on his face and from under his jacket he pulled out a soft, white ball of fluff. It was a tiny little kitten that I named "Snowball." He was precious — so frisky and so beautiful with his long, silky fur and gold-green eyes.

We bonded almost instantly. Snowball followed me everywhere during the day and slept with me at night. He lay on the kitchen counter when I cooked or did the dishes. He sat on the bathroom counter when I put on my makeup and did my hair. When I came home from work he would always be waiting at the window and he would greet me with a meow, his beautiful fluffy tail standing straight up like a flag of welcome. I talked to him like he was a person and he talked back to me too. I learned which meow meant "I'm hungry" and which meant "pet me" and "play with me." He would actually check out the different men I dated over the years and he'd let me know which ones he thought were not acceptable by hissing at them. In every way, he was a close companion, he gave purpose to my life and we loved each other.

When Snowball was a year old, I thought he might be lonely while I was at work so I got another kitten to be his companion. At first Snowball made life hard for poor Inky. He let Inky know that he was Number One Kitty. Once Inky accepted his place as second kitty, Snowball stopped harassing him.

I dated a doctor for several years but when he finished his residency he decided to leave because he said that he didn't want to be tied down. I was devastated. I lost 25 pounds. I couldn't eat or sleep and I wanted to die. During this bad time Snowball seemed to sense that I was sad and he would follow me everywhere I went. It seemed as if he was trying to comfort me. Inky was much more aloof and independent; he was not a "people cat."

I was in the depths of despair. One day I sat

crying in the bathroom with a full bottle of sleeping pills in one hand and a big glass of water in the other. I was determined to end my pain once and for all. Snowball came into the bathroom, sat at my feet, rubbed against my legs and meowed loudly. I was in too much despair to pay attention to him.

Then a miracle happened. Snowball jumped on my lap. He looked in my face and meowed as if he was asking me, "What's wrong?" With one white paw he touched my tear-stained cheek and then licked a tear off my face. Suddenly I became aware of what I was doing and I put down the pills. I knew I couldn't leave Snowball — he needed me.

My cat really seemed to know what I was feeling and he found a way to tell me that he loved me. I cried and hugged Snowball for a long time, knowing he had saved my life.

I called my mom and she helped me find a therapist. After some months of therapy, I became myself again. Snowball and I were even closer after that. He was protective of me and never left my side when I was home. Our bond of love grew stronger.

I then fell in love with a man and we were married one year later on New Year's Eve. Snowball liked him too. We all moved to a rural area south of Tucson where my new husband lived on six acres of land. He had two cats of his own. At first, there was a lot of jealousy between the four cats, but as soon as the other cats agreed that Snowball was Number One, they all got along. We were a very happy family.

Two years later Snowball began to lose weight, his fur lost its luster and he seemed lethargic. I took him to the vet and spent a fortune on diagnostic tests. When the results came in we found out that Snowball had diabetes. I had to bring him to the hospital every day for a week so that he could get started on insulin and a new diet.

    I lived in fear that he would not recover, that he would die. My friends told me to have him put to sleep, but that seemed so cruel; also, he was my sweet baby and had saved my life. I was determined to do everything possible to save him.

    I learned to give Snowball an insulin injection every morning and how to test his urine for sugar. Being a nurse helped; I was familiar with giving injections and watching for signs of trouble. As time passed Snowball gained weight and he started to play again. Again he followed me everywhere. As if we both knew that our time together was limited, our love became stronger. I lived in constant fear that I would come home from work one day and find him sick, but thankfully he continued to thrive. We settled into a routine, but I was always afraid.

    Two years later my husband and I went to visit his parents in the White Mountains of Arizona. Because he hated to be boarded at the vet's, I decided to take Snowball with me. I packed his insulin and syringes and away we went. We had a wonderful time! Snowball loved the pine trees and the coolness of the woods. We took some great photographs of Snowball. It was a special time for us.

    Recently my husband and I decided to go camping for a couple of days in the mountains near our home. It was too hot to take Snowball with us so he had to stay behind. I hated to board him and I knew he hated it, but I had been working overtime and needed to get away. The whole time we were away I worried about Snowball.

Monday afternoon I eagerly drove to the vet's to pick up Snowball. When I got him home he didn't seem to be his normal self. By early Tuesday morning, I knew he was sick. I called the vet and raced him in. She said he was in serious trouble. I left him so she could draw blood, do x-rays and run tests. I returned to pick him up a few hours later. My poor baby was so weak he could barely walk, but he meowed when he saw me and lifted his fluffy tail up briefly, then lay quietly in my lap. The vet didn't know what was wrong; his x-rays and blood sugar were normal, but we still had to wait for the lab results. I took him home, held him, prayed for him and cried all afternoon. When my husband came home from work I told him, "Snowball is dying." We cried together.

Snowball could not eat or drink and he vomited a few times. His breathing was labored, but he still wanted to be near me — he lay beside me on the couch and then on my lap. That night, he snuggled up to me, put his soft paw on my cheek and looked into my face with his beautiful gold-green eyes, now dilated with approaching death. He meowed softly and I knew he was saying "I love you." I think he knew he was dying. We stayed that way for awhile. Then he crawled off my lap and tried to jump to the floor, but he couldn't. I gently placed him on the floor. He tried to walk, but was too weak, so I helped him by supporting his weight. He went into the bathroom and lay down next to the tub where he often sat while I was taking a shower. We sat there in the dark. He lay with his head supported on my hand while I stroked him and told him I loved him, that he was my sweet baby, that I would never forget him and that one day we would be together again. I prayed for him over and over and I cried. My husband joined me and the three of us stayed there in the dark.

Snowball looked into my eyes again and meowed. He turned around so his face and head were back against the wall. I knew the end was near — his breathing was ragged and irregular. From time to time he meowed — a sad, mournful sound that seemed to come from his soul, a cry of anguish that broke my heart.

I went to the phone and called the vet at home to see if there was anything I could do to ease his pain. While I was on the phone, my husband called to me, "He's going." He was crying, too. Snowball breathed his last breath at 9:30 p.m. He was ten days short of his ninth birthday.

I brushed him one more time. (He loved to be brushed. Whenever I combed my hair, Snowball was there to get his hair combed too.) I wrapped him in his favorite sheepskin blanket and held him all night. I talked to him and I cried and prayed. I watched the sun rise with my sweet baby in my arms.

My husband dug a grave under a mesquite tree in the back of our property where there is a great view of the mountains. We buried Snowball next to my husband's dog who had died before I met him.

I put pretty sparkling rocks and a red rose from my garden on Snowball's grave. I also put a brown cross on his grave that had hung on my wall as a child. I said goodbye to my baby.

The next day I went to work and told my friends what had happened. They were sympathetic, but also seemed not to understand my pain. They looked at me and I knew they were thinking, "It's only a cat. Why is she so upset?"

The vet said that Snowball had died of kidney and liver failure — a complication caused by the diabetes — and that there was nothing we could have done to save him. But I am not comforted. I am *angry* that he was taken from me. I'm *angry* that my friends don't understand my pain. I am heartsick in my grief. I feel as if I have died inside. Only my husband understands and comforts me and I am grateful for his support. He went through the same thing with his dog so he understands how I feel.

In the morning before work I go to Snowball's grave to talk to him and cry for him. In the evening I put a rose on his grave. I tell him, "Snowball, I love you. You will always be with me in spirit." I tell him about my day and how I miss him. I talk as if he can hear me and I believe he can. I tell him we *will* be together again someday. I spend a lot of time at his grave. Each night we watch the sun set. I miss my sweet baby, my little love, so very, very much.

My work is to comfort the sick and the dying and Snowball's death has only increased my compassion for the patients I care for and their families. I now know firsthand what they feel — the loss and the pain.

We are told that "time heals all" and I guess my pain will lessen with time and my grief will become bearable. But I am suffering now. I miss Snowball so much. My heart aches with a physical pain that only one who has lost a loved one can understand. Despite the pain, I am so thankful that Snowball was a part of my life.

The ancient Egyptians believed that to speak the name of the dead is to make them live again and I agree. It will comfort me to know that

Snowball's memory will live on in your book. More than that, I hope my story will help others understand that it is normal to grieve for the loss of a beloved pet.

Sincerely,

L.S., Arizona

The Cat Who Died for Me

Dear Kymberly,

For the first time in five years, I am very lonely. That is the date on which Fluffo and I became close. Now she is gone and I miss her so...
    I will tell you what happened to her, but first I want to tell you what Fluffo meant to me. She was my companion, my family, the only one in the world who loved and nurtured me. She took the despair out of my life, she gave me the strength to make very difficult decisions, she eased my pain. She made me feel important and wanted.
    My life centered around Fluffo. My heart felt safe loving her. I gave her a lot and she had repaid me with interest a million times over. Whenever I thought of the future, she was part of my plans. In a word, she inspired me.
    Fluffo's happiness was my first concern. Once she was sitting peacefully on my lap. When a friend sat down, Fluffo left my lap for my friend's. My friend was flattered — rightfully so. At first, I must admit, I felt somewhat hurt. But then I thought: If this is the way Fluffo is happier, then I am happy too. My friend said: "All you care about is Fluffo's

happiness."

There came a time when I had to be away from Fluffo for an extended period and I had to leave her with a caretaker. Apparently, every day Fluffo waited for my return — patiently, trustfully and hopefully. Whenever she heard my voice over the telephone, she would meow and purr to me. But one day she didn't hear my voice anymore. When I called, her caretaker — a person I thought was my friend — began to do something that to this day I cannot understand: she wouldn't let me talk to Fluffo. Time passed and eventually Fluffo must have concluded that I was gone for good, that I would never return. I have now been able to reconstruct the scenario of Fluffo's last months, and I can say — without much fear of being mistaken — that Fluffo committed suicide.

Fluffo starved herself to death. She was not sick and there was no other reason for her to stop eating except for sadness over my disappearance. Her caretaker had always assured me over the phone that she was all right, but clearly she didn't watch carefully and she didn't realize that Fluffo was acting differently — or she did and didn't care.

Fluffo died because she loved me, because I was the only being who understood, respected and loved her — the only one who bothered to reach out to her, to listen to her and to respond to her needs. Fluffo died *for me*. She died of grief. She let me know this by dying just two days short of the very month and day when, exactly a year before, I had left her. I believe her plan was to die on the anniversary date, but she was so weakened by lack of nourishment that, in all likelihood, the run-in she had with another cat may have hastened her end.

Once I was privileged enough to quietly accept that Fluffo was happier on someone else's lap, even if it hurt my feelings. But just as Fluffo's happiness mattered most to me then, it is now Fluffo's suffering that matters most to me.

I think about the pain that she must have endured during those long months that she waited for me in vain, when she had questions and no one was there to answer them. I think about her inability to understand my absence and about her feelings of abandonment, betrayal, loneliness and despair. She had put her trust in me. She had relied on me and was unjustly punished. I can see her now, each day eagerly awaiting my return home, just as I had returned so often before. And each day her hopes were dashed. How cruel I had been to her, albeit unknowingly. And how unimportant my pain is compared to hers. Fluffo is truly "The Cat Who Died for Me." My punishment is that she took away what was most dear to me.

It has been very helpful for me to write about this terrible experience. I hope it will make other people who may read my letter understand that cats can have feelings very much like people. They can feel the pain of abandonment so intensely that they don't want to live anymore. Therefore no one should make the mistake of thinking that animals don't get depressed.

Sincerely,

E.T.H., New York

A Mother Cat Mourns

Dear Kymberly,

I want to tell you a touching story about my personal experience with death with the hope that it might help others who read it.

One summer a remarkable cat padded into my life. She simply appeared at my door one day — timid, frightened and indescribably beautiful. Less than a year old, she looked like an ocelot wearing socks with her brown-gray, whorl-patterned tabby and white coat. After befriending my male Siamese cat, Vlad, she began spending more and more time around my house. I had a suspicion that she had been abandoned by someone living in the apartments across the street. Our neighborhood is filled with cats that have been abandoned by transient families. They often purchase kittens for their children and when the time comes to move, the unaltered animals are left behind to fend for themselves.

A few weeks after the cat's arrival, my father and I decided to mow the lawn and clean up our front yard. Looking through our chaotic garage for garden tools, I heard the tiniest sound, like a squeak toy. Investigating the source of the sound, I discovered a box containing three tiny kittens that all looked like ocelots wearing socks.

My joy was indescribable. I cherished them like they were my own children. Until then, I had only seen newborn kittens in pictures and on television. In the midst of my joy the mother cat returned to her little ones, picking each up by its scruff and moving it away from me. It took some doing, but I persuaded her to bed them down in a cleaner box without potentially dangerous sharp objects lurking in it. Convinced that she had no owners, my father and I resolved to adopt "Mama Cat."

The next few days were the happiest of my life. My thoughts were full of kittens. After work I would rush home to see them, to hold their tiny bodies in my hands. Mama Cat trusted me more and more, and didn't mind my intrusions. But my happiness didn't last long.

The first sadness happened three days after I discovered the kittens. My father called me at work and told me that the smallest of the three was dead, though he didn't know why. For some reason, I wasn't terribly upset. I guess I understood that sometimes the weakest kittens die to make way for the stronger ones. That night I placed the kitten's dead body in a paper bag, ready for a proper burial the next day. I gently touched the two living kittens, trying to think of names for them, imagining how beautiful they would be as adults. On my calendar, I marked the milestone days to come — when I could feed the kittens milk and soft food, when their eyes would open, when they would start walking.

I went to work the following day full of hope

and happiness. It was early evening when I got home. Still in my dress clothes, I tiptoed into the garage and sat down on a box near Mama Cat and her little ones. Not looking into the box, I spoke softly to the frightened cat, assuring her that I meant no harm to her or her children. Suddenly, I realized that there were no sounds coming from the box. Leaping to my feet, I looked with horror at the cold, stiffening bodies of the two kittens. Mama Cat, confused, kept lying on her side and pushing them against her swollen teats, trying to nurse them. I screamed, then sobbed and ran from the garage. I ran out to the sidewalk and just kept running until my legs hurt.

When I buried the kittens, I was not the same person I was when I discovered them alive and well only days before. I had become a person without hope. Packing the earth over the tiny parcel, I gazed blankly at the bleak sky and wondered what kind of God would take the lives of these innocent creatures. Why are lives brought into this world only to be quickly and mercilessly snatched away? My grief, like my earlier joy, was indescribable.

It is the way of animals to focus on the living. When animals lose a loved one, they tend to put all their energy into caring for the other remaining loved ones. With this thought in mind, I drove out to the local humane society and adopted two black male kittens, brothers whom I immediately named Heckle and Jeckle after the cartoon characters. From the start they were two bundles of renewed hope. Playful and demanding, they left me with little time for grief. Mama Cat, always the caregiver, treated them as if they were her own — washing them, teaching them how to hunt mice and insects and generally keeping them in line.

For about six months all went well. Heckle turned out to be the bigger and more affectionate of the two, with a loud voice and a boisterous personality. Smaller and quieter, Jeckle would occasionally sit in my lap, but mostly he wanted to be left alone. I loved him all the more because of this. I admired his strange, penetrating eyes and wondered what he was thinking as he sat for hours staring into space. I gave him extra attention, thinking that perhaps he felt left out in a four-cat household. And then he got sick.

At first, I wasn't sure which cat was sick; I only found pools of vomit on the floor. I thought that one of them had eaten something bad from the garbage and had simply been nauseous. I never suspected a serious illness. The next night, Jeckle vomited up a foul-smelling green substance and he seemed to be in pain. He seemed not to know where he was or what was happening. I still curse myself for failing to call the emergency vet. I don't know if it would have made any difference, but we always blame ourselves for the tragic things that happen to our loved ones.

During the night, Jeckle's spirit left his body and somehow I knew it. There was something missing from the house. I didn't want to get out of bed. If I don't get up, I thought, it won't have happened. Maybe if I go back to sleep, I'll wake up to a different outcome.

Mama Cat mourned the loss of Jeckle relentlessly and for several weeks after his death, she ran frantically through the house and garage, looking for him, calling him. When she realized that he was gone, she wailed all night in grief. She would jump up on my bed in the middle of the night, awaking me with a start, and look desperately into my eyes. Her pitiful crying would make me start to cry as well. I wondered why life had cheated her so, taking away her own kittens in their infancy, then allowing her to adopt and love another kitten before he too was snatched away.

Immediately after Jeckle's death, I was forced to focus on the living. I could see that Heckle was also sick with the same illness because he was displaying the same signs. I rushed him to the vet and thankfully, he survived. I can still see my father holding Heckle in the vet's examination room, looking deeply into his eyes and saying "Please don't die, please don't die" over and over again.

Mama and Heckle have become the best of friends. Old Vlad is a bit jealous, but he still commands plenty of Mama's attention. We go on living; what choice do we have? For one thing, these experiences made me think about how cruel it is that people hunt and kill wild animals and I wondered whether they grieve when they lose their companions and family members to the trap or the gun. It's time we started giving animals more respect. I learned from Mama Cat that they have feelings just like people.

Sincerely,

B.W., California

Death by Negligence?

Dear Kymberly,

We are emigrants from Bucharest, Romania. My husband came to New York two years ago and I followed one year later. I have a sad story to tell you.
    My flight from Bucharest to New York was lovely because I traveled with my beloved four-year-old cat, Ionut. His coat was spotted white and brown, his eyes were blue, and he had a gorgeous tail. Some of my family and friends told me that I was really crazy to take Ionut to New York, but it was impossible for me to leave him behind. I couldn't live without him and I don't think he could live without me. I wasn't about to betray him. Moreover, my husband had missed Ionut and was looking forward to his arrival in New York.
    My husband met us at JFK Airport and we were glad to be together again. Ionut and I were tired after 12 hours of flying and my husband had been waiting, very excited, for four hours. I told him that during the journey Ionut had been so good, quiet and gentle. Many people on the plane wanted to look at him and touch him. I was so

proud of my adorable cat. My husband took the cat in his arms and caressed him with love, but it seemed Ionut didn't recognize him. This saddened my husband.

In the car, Ionut looked at me with his beautiful blue eyes for a long time. It seemed he was asking me "Where are we now? Where are we going? What has happened to us?" I wish I could have explained that the three of us were going to start a new life in a little apartment in a new country, very different from our Romanian life. To my surprise, Ionut became accustomed quite fast to New York. I think he liked American food.

Because Ionut was always a very curious cat, he wanted to know about everything around him. He liked to climb in the wardrobe, to run throughout the apartment and to look out the window and sit on the balcony. We played together every day. Sometimes he would go to our neighbor's door, looking, I think, for our former five-year-old neighbor in Bucharest. She was his closest friend besides my husband and I. Ionut walked upstairs and downstairs because he had this habit in Bucharest. At times he became scared and meowed terribly, maybe because he couldn't find the places he used to know.

After two months, we had to move because our landlord didn't like cats. Immediately Ionut had to inspect everything in the new apartment. At first he was sad, anxious and scared and we had to help him regain his composure and cheerfulness, but in time, he became himself — well-balanced, joyful and frolicsome. Our new apartment was larger than the first and Ionut enjoyed running through the rooms. Ionut liked to be combed, spoiled and to sleep in my lap or in my bed. When we would come home, Ionut would be waiting at the door.

About five months later something suddenly seemed wrong with Ionut. He ate very little and he couldn't jump and run as usual. He didn't like to play with us or with his toys and he looked tired. My husband and I were worried and we hoped it wasn't serious. I made an appointment for him at the local animal hospital and two doctors examined Ionut and told us that he had an infection in his mouth, but that he could be treated. They assured us that our cat would be okay. Although the cost of treatment was a lot for us at that time, we agreed. We wanted to stay at the hospital during the treatment, but the doctors would not allow it. When we left, Ionut just looked at us helplessly.

About two hours later, somebody called us from the animal hospital, saying something confusing about an accident and that I should come as soon as possible. I immediately told my husband. Because I was starting to get upset, he tried to assure me that I probably misunderstood the message. "Don't worry," he said, "you will see everything will be all right, believe me."

When we got to the hospital, my husband went into the examination room. After a few minutes he came out crying and he took me inside. On the table lay Ionut. He was dead.

When I saw my poor cat, I lost control. My husband caught me in time because I would have fallen to the floor. We cried together. We looked at Ionut, caressed him and cried some more. We spoke to him in Romanian and in English. The doctors tried to tell us that our cat died because he couldn't handle the anesthesia, but we didn't believe them.

We stayed with Ionut for about an hour. I

asked God to punish the doctors and to take me as well. My heart was broken and I hoped that I would die. We wanted to take our dead cat with us but the doctors wouldn't allow it. Finally, we agreed that he should be cremated.

I got sick and stayed in bed for five days without eating. I mourned for my beloved cat. My husband tried to console me and stayed home with me instead of going to work. I recovered for a while, but I got sick again. It is a very long story, impossible for me to describe in a few pages.

I'll never forget my cat, Ionut. My husband and I still cry when we think about him. His ashes that we keep in a box and his toys are our treasures.

I wrote to the animal hospital two times asking for an explanation about the death of our cat, but I never received an answer. In my eyes the doctors there are guilty; they are responsible for the death of my beloved Ionut. I am sure they care for animals only for the money they can make. In my opinion, it's only business to them.

Very truly yours,

F.U., New York

Telepathy

Dear Kymberly,

As I write this letter, I am 64 years old. Thirteen years ago, my teenage daughter brought home a calico kitten. Because my wife worked and I was the "house husband," I somehow knew that despite all my family's promises, most of the responsibility for caring for this cat would be mine. We debated the pros and cons of keeping the cat and finally decided to take a vote. I cast the only dissenting vote; the kitten was here to stay. Her name was Bear, short for Wooley Bear.

Two months ago — thirteen years later — we were faced with making another decision concerning Bear — but this time it was a sad decision. Even though she was a house cat and was never outside except when tethered to the house, she had somehow contracted infectious peritonitis. Her last month with us was just awful. As she became sicker, she had more and more difficulty eating and her breathing sounded as though she had something caught in her throat. After almost a week in the hospital, we knew something had to be done. This time the decision was all mine. Bear — my Bear by this time — would have to be put to sleep.

It's been two months since I took Bear to the vet for the last time. I'm still grieving. I miss my kitty and the tears come easily when I look at her photo over my desk or when I hug my dalmatian.

At first, Bear and I were not the best of friends. She was an intruder, an interruption in my life. In time, however, a bond began to form between us. She was a terror in the kitchen, jumping from object to object, climbing the drapes with her claws. I would chase her all over the house, hollering and throwing things. Still, even after all of my shameful abuse, she would crawl onto my chest and lay there with her face against mine.

She was not an overly affectionate cat and would hiss at any advances from my wife and daughters. But she and I had something special going. I was always the one she favored. I understood her and she understood me. There was a telepathy between us that did not exist between her and the other members of the family. I knew when she wanted to go out and when she was sitting silently at the front door waiting to be let in. When I opened the front door and whistled or called for her to come in, she would immediately come running.

I am not ashamed to say that for about two weeks after Bear was put to sleep, I was in a very bad way. Tears from a 64-year-old man are not much appreciated or understood by some people, especially when they are for a dead cat. And so I tried to repress the grief I felt. I also started to feel a lot of guilt and wondered if I had put Bear to sleep because I could no longer deal with her suffering. Listening to her trying to breathe and trying unsuccessfully to eat hurt me so much. I told my vet about this guilt and he gave me a pamphlet about dealing with issues of guilt and this helped me to overcome some of these feelings.

Nevertheless, I still missed Bear terribly. I couldn't even look at a photograph of her without crying. I tried putting the photo away, but then decided that it was not fair to Bear. Holding in my feelings began to affect my health. I couldn't sleep because I had developed severe stomach pains. I spent days just lying in bed. Then one day, as I sat sorting through photos, all my repressed feelings broke loose and I let myself cry for a while. That night I was finally able to sleep without pain.

Another bit of torture I put myself through was asking the vet how they had disposed of Bear's body. Unfortunately, when they originally asked me if I wanted to take her body with me, I declined. I was far too upset to carry her dead body home. I also believed, for some naive reason, that the animal hospital would do something decent and respectable with Bear's body. Instead, Bear was picked up and taken to the city landfill, only to be pushed around by a bulldozer like a clump of garbage.

One other thing that bothered me was a theological question. Had God made provisions for domesticated animals? As a Christian I understood that God had made us different from animals. As humans, we have a soul and the presence of His Holy Spirit within us. However, if God was concerned and aware enough to know when a sparrow fell, I can only believe that He takes care of animals after they die, that he'd never allow His creatures to fall away into nothingness. I am, therefore, counting on seeing my Bear again.

R.F., Washington

The Disappeared

Dear Kymberly,

One thought I can't get out of my head is that I *should have known* that something was wrong. Instead, I sat there totally absorbed in the movie I was watching while my Augustus jumped out an open window and disappeared into the night. I didn't even notice. Why didn't I get a message? I loved him so much, I would have thought that our psychic bond would have alerted me. Maybe I just didn't hear him call to me. I know he must have been scared.

    I never let my cats outside. Especially for city dwellers, the outside world can be a dangerous place. And what would have made it even more terrifying for Augustus was that nothing would be familiar. I don't know if I had ever felt as guilty in my life....

    It was not the best of times for me: I lost my father to a stroke, went through a divorce, changed jobs, moved to a new place and was caring for a sick brother. But no one believes me when I tell them that losing Gusser was the most traumatic event of all for me. I was told that my grief was "misplaced," that I was burying my "real" pain by talking about Augustus.

How I craved a sympathetic word from someone — anyone — about my feelings for Augustus. The one time that my uncle told me he could appreciate my love for my cat and the pain I was feeling about his disappearance, the words seemed like manna from heaven. I couldn't get over how much it meant to have my feelings for Augustus acknowledged.

I put ads in the paper to see if anyone had seen or found him. I went through the roller coaster ride of expectation whenever a call came in, only to be cruelly disappointed each time. I searched the streets day and night, put up posters, visited the animal shelters (which was a painful act in itself) and offered rewards. Nothing came through. Once, in the pound, I saw their listing of dead animals that had been found and one of them sounded like Augustus. I asked if I could see him, but the woman patted my hand and said that it would be too traumatic for me to see the dead animals. She talked me out of it and to this day I regret it. At least, if the dead cat had been Gusser, I would have known. On the other hand, maybe the woman was right; maybe it would have been too upsetting to see.

Not knowing was the worst. The mind can come up with all kinds of images, some of them terrible. At first there was a glimmer of hope that someone took him in and was loving him, but then my mind would drift toward the negative. Maybe I just wanted to torture myself for being so irresponsible; maybe I was seeking some kind of punishment or atonement.

If only he could hear me, I know what I'd

say: "I'm so sorry, Augustus. I miss you so much. I hope with all my heart that you weren't scared, that you were rescued from the streets. I'm sorry I got mad at you when you didn't come home. I thought maybe you didn't love me. I've read about animals who journey hundreds of miles to be reunited with their family, seemingly driven only by love, and I want the same for us. I do feel I let you down." If only I had shut the window....

K.A., California

My Feline Children

Dear Kymberly,

I heard about the book you were writing and I thought you might like to hear my story.

I am a middle-aged, divorced man with no human children, but I do have 16 feline children. In the past two years, I have lost three cats and I'm afraid that another one is dying now. Before I tell you about these dear companions, please understand that I am a very caring person who looks on each cat as one of my children, even the three feral cats that have come to live with me.

The first cat I lost was Wadsworth. He suddenly became listless and his fur got shabby. My vet assured me that he wasn't in pain, but Wadsworth was only a year and a half old and I needed some sort of explanation. I took him to the local animal clinic and he was scheduled for a series of tests. While he was struggling to avoid being x-rayed, Wadsworth's heart gave out; an autopsy showed that he had cancer of the lymph nodes.

Smokey, my 10-year-old gray female, went from frisky to barely moving in only 48 hours. It didn't take the vet long to see that her liver was badly diseased. There was nothing to do but put her to sleep. Smokey was my number one lap cat and her purr could fill a room. I cried all night after her death.

Just three weeks ago, my adorable five-month-old kitten, Fluffernutter, died of pneumonia. I had taken him to the vet only the day before. He was given a shot and he seemed to improve almost immediately. I came home from work the next night and Fluffernutter was nowhere to be found. After searching the house, I finally discovered him dead in the litter box. He was an orange long-hair and a real love.

Now I'm watching Blackie, my black male, as he wastes away. Blackie has the best personality of any cat I've ever known. Even my other cats won't fight or argue with him. He gets along with all of them. Even people who don't like cats like him. Blackie tested positive for feline leukemia four years ago so I've been watching him closely. My vet recently diagnosed him as anemic. He's given Blackie liver and vitamin shots and given me pills to give as well, but I can't get him to eat. I don't want to have to resort to force-feeding Blackie, but I'm not sure that I have any choice.

What hurts me most is that after each of the deaths, people would say things like "Well, you've got plenty more" or "That's one less to feed." People who aren't animal lovers don't seem to realize how much it hurts to lose a pet, no matter how large your family may be. Each one is a true individual with a distinct personality and a unique set of qualities. No one would dream of dismissing the death of a human child from a big family in that way. And yet when someone loses a beloved animal companion, the number of other family members is thought to reduce the pain.

Sincerely,

L.S., Illinois

A Big, Empty Spot

Dear Kymberly,

I am 12 years old and I want to tell you my story. Last November we adopted a cat. I named her Apple-bee after a friend's cat who died. My family was about to move and I was worried about how that would affect Apple-bee, especially since our new house was right on a highway. I was worried that she would get run over or stolen.

One of the first things we did after moving was to take her to the vet to give her a check-up and have her spayed. When Apple-bee turned two the following March, the vet sent her a birthday card.

At first, Apple-bee loved to go outside — whenever she wasn't eating. But even though she ate and ate, she never got fat. We even asked the vet to check to see if she had worms, but she didn't. I became concerned when Apple-bee started staying inside most of the time. I thought it was strange for a cat who loved the outside. Even when she needed to go out, she wouldn't, so I finally had to make her go outside. The next day, Apple-bee didn't come home for breakfast. I knew something was very wrong — Apple-bee would never miss a meal. But I didn't give up hope. I searched in every place I could think of. I made signs and hung them up around town. It didn't help. Still, I looked and looked and cried and cried. Nothing worked. Apple-bee never came home. I blame it on myself because I made her go outside.

Last month, I saw an article in a magazine about whether cats are psychic. It got me thinking: Maybe Apple-bee knew that something was going to happen to her if she went outside. Maybe that is why she tried so hard to stay inside.

Now I have only my memories of Apple-bee. She was a bossy cat, but I loved her more than anything. Also, she couldn't stand to wait for her food. If my mom wasn't up by 5:30 to feed her, she would wake her up. The one thing that Apple-bee didn't like was expensive cat food, she liked the Alpo brand. She was warm and cuddly and very, very pretty.

My mom loved Apple-bee, too. She didn't like the name. In fact, everyone picked on me about her name, but I liked it. She was an odd cat so she needed an odd name. When Apple-bee disappeared, my mom may not have cried out loud but she cried on the inside. Losing Apple-bee left a big, empty spot in our hearts.

Sincerely,

C.S., Louisiana

Puppyraisers

Dear Kymberly,

There is a category relating to pet loss that I think many people overlook. It is similar to the loss experienced when a pet dies, in that there is a forced separation, but it is also very different because the animal is still alive.

    Everyone knows about guide dogs for the blind, signal or hearing dogs for the deaf and service dogs for the physically challenged. What many people never think about is that there is a puppyraiser who cared for and loved each one of these dogs — from the time he (or she) was eight or nine weeks old until he was 16 to 20 months old — and then had to give him up.

    There are several things that make the separation that a puppyraiser experiences different from other types of loss. While people always talk about what a wonderful thing a puppyraiser is doing, I often feel that they are also thinking something else — "You are doing such a wonderful thing, but of course *I* could never do it. I love my animals too much to ever give one up." The inference is that if puppyraisers really loved their animals, they couldn't part with them and that they must be cold people to be able to do this. As a result, when the time to part comes around, some people do not quite know how to react to my feelings of loss. After all, they think, because I am a puppyraiser, I knew I would eventually give the dog up. Puppyraisers who mourn the parting (in other words, the loss) of a dog get very little support even from friends who would otherwise be supportive if a pet were to die.

What they do not understand is that the grief breeders feel when they give up a pet is every bit as real and deep as the grief that results from the death of a pet. When I returned home from "turning in" my first puppy, I was alone with my grief. I knew I had support from other puppyraisers and service dog recipients, but these people were acquaintances at best; my friends and family didn't know how to react and didn't understand the depth of my feelings.

Each year there are hundreds of us puppyraisers who are experiencing the pain of loss of a beloved "foster child." We do not love our animals less, we love our fellow man more. We, too, need help, understanding and support when we say goodbye.

In an effort to walk through the grief I felt after I said my goodbyes to one dog I raised, Oski, I wrote my feelings down. This is what I wrote:

A Farewell to Oski

An unfamiliar sense of quiet permeates the atmosphere in my home tonight. I hold the needlepoint pillow with one corner missing and am amazed to realize that I am glad Oski chewed it. A solitary tear winds its way down my cheek as my fingers travel back and forth over the frayed edges and I know that I will always treasure this piece of tangible evidence that for a brief 15 months, an incredibly complex, intelligent, exuberant, affectionate, sometimes naughty and altogether wonderful border collie named Oski lit up my life and my dog Alice's life, too.

  He is gone now. This morning Alice and I drove him to the training center, a beautiful place in the country. Together we explored the grounds. Oski was fascinated with the ducks, chickens, goats, horses and sheep. We placed a ball in the exercise yard and Alice left her scent to comfort him in the difficult days to come. When we were finished playing, we went into the kennels. Alice and Oski charged into the run that was to be Oski's and quenched their thirst from the water dish. I told him that this was his home now.

  After our tour, we went to the office where his new trainer was waiting for us. She hugged me and said that it was time to say goodbye. I watched him happily walk off with her, his tail gaily wagging and I knew that she had been right when she said that it would be easier for him to leave me than for him to watch me walk away. Alice and I turned and left. We did not look back.

  Oh, Oski, I love you so deeply! I will miss you more than you could ever understand. Be a good boy. Adjust to your new life. Learn well and be happy. Make me proud. You are a very special dog, born and raised for a very special purpose. Farewell, my friend. I shall never forget you.

  I want to add that there are rewards for doing what puppyraisers do. Oski became a signal dog for a deaf couple. He has been on television several times helping to enhance public awareness of the function he serves. The deaf couple has recently become the parents of twin babies and Oski's ears are the only ears in that home to hear the babies' cries and to alert the parents that the babies require attention. In 1990, Oski was a nominee for the Delta Society's Support Dog of the Year award. I am very proud of him.

Sincerely,

P.W., California

A Dog's Courage

Dear Kymberly,

In 1976 I was diagnosed with multiple sclerosis. Among the do's and don't's I received from the doctor was that I should not get a dog. How strange, I thought, to specifically rule out dogs when the cause and cure of the disease were still unknown and certainly didn't have anything to do with dogs. At that time, my husband and I had been married for seven years and we had no children. I was also advised not to get pregnant and have children.

    I wanted to listen to the doctor's advice, but on the day I saw Smokey, I simply couldn't resist. She was the most perfect little puppy and from the moment I picked her up and held her, I fell in love. The bond that we developed with Smokey became stronger and stronger. Soon, I couldn't imagine life without her.

    Smokey was a shepherd mix, extremely loyal and always ready to please. She learned quickly. Just as soon as she was big enough, she would retrieve the newspaper and this became a daily job. She would be so anxious to fetch the paper that she would wake us up on weekends at four in the morning so she could get it.

    My parents live right behind us and I would have Smokey take things over to them and she would bring things from them back to me. One spring day I was out cleaning the yard and my father commented, "You teach this dog everything else, why don't you teach her how to use the toilet?" I didn't pay much attention and put the thought out of my head. The next morning I noticed that the carpet in the bathroom was wet and told my husband that the toilet was leaking. We dried the area and waited to see where it was leaking from. A few hours later we noticed that the water was yellow and I realized that Smokey had created this "leak." I talked to Smokey and told her that she was a good girl but if she had to go potty, she should go outside. She knew what the bathroom was for, just not quite how to use it. Had she actually understood what my father had said? I believe she did. There are many stories I could tell you that you wouldn't believe.

    I think you can understand that Smokey was more than just smart. She was also obedient and she never did anything that would cause us to reprimand her. She was just about perfect.

    Then after 12 years we began to notice that Smokey seemed a little disoriented while she was doing the most routine things. She'd go outside to get the paper and after going half way she'd turn around and look at us as if to say, "What was I about to do?" That was the beginning of the battle.

    I took her to the vet and learned that she had possible lymphosarcoma (cancer of the lymph glands). I was in such shock while driving home that I had to pull over to calm down. By the time I got home I was crying so hard that I could hardly tell my husband what had happened. Whenever someone would ask about Smokey, I burst into tears.

During the last six months of Smokey's life we did everything humanly possible to keep her alive. She was started on weekly chemotherapy and even though it made her very sick, she never stopped wanting to please us. Each week there was a new problem and it got harder and harder for us to manage. During her last three weeks she began choking. The cancer had spread to her lungs. There are no words to describe the fear that overtook us when we realized that we were losing the battle. We could not even imagine not having Smokey with us.

On the morning of her birthday, we took Smokey to the vet for what turned out to be the last time. My husband had evidently made up his mind that we couldn't let her suffer anymore and that we had to put her out of her misery. The vet discussed euthanasia with us in a kind and calming way. Even though we agreed that it was the only humane thing to do, I couldn't believe my ears when I heard my husband say, through his tears, "If it's necessary, then do it."

Neither of us could bear to be there for the injection. We visited a pet cemetery and made the needed arrangements. I asked them to wait one night before burying her so I could get all of her toys together so they could be buried with her.

Coming home without Smokey was excruciatingly painful. The cake mix that I had taken out that morning was still on the counter. I looked at her toys and her food and water dishes and felt miserable. The next morning I had to walk outside and get the paper myself — it was the first time in

13 years. There was the worst empty feeling in my heart and home. Telling people what happened was more painful than words can describe.

As I write this, more than three years later, the tears and hurt have welled up all over again. To this day I go to the cemetery once a week to visit Smokey. I talk out loud to her and clean off her tombstone. It is of some comfort knowing that we did everything humanly possible for her, but I miss her terribly.

After we lost Smokey, my husband and I decided to get another dog. After traveling all over the state looking for the right one, not just a "replacement," we finally chose a little yorkie-poo. When we brought her home, my mother wouldn't even look at her because she never again wanted to become attached to an animal and then lose her. We love our new dog very much, but she is not Smokey and never will be.

I made a collage with some of Smokey's pictures and I hung it right next to my bed so I can look at her each morning. Crazy as it may seem, I still talk to her as if she's right here. She was always such a comfort lying so close to me when I was sleeping or sick. I think that it really helps to be able to talk about your loss with someone who is a dog lover or who has gone through a similar experience. Visiting her gravestone weekly to tell her what's been going on and talking with others has helped somewhat, but the deep pain still remains.

Neither my husband nor I have ever experienced a greater loss than Smokey's. Relatives have died but it's different because we were not responsible for their welfare and they were not as close to us as Smokey was. People say, "But she was just a dog!" Not Smokey; she was human in ways they can't imagine unless they've been fortunate enough to have such a friend. I do believe that it is better to have loved and lost than never to have loved at all. I must remember my faith and know that God has Smokey in a place that is free from all pain. Smokey was totally courageous as she faced her final battle. She taught me so much.

    I don't know if it was fair to our new pet to have gotten her so soon after Smokey's death, but I just had to have another "baby" close to me. It felt good trying to keep up with such an obstinate, exuberant puppy until she would have an accident and that made me remember how different Smokey was.

    If there is an easy way to sort through the flood of emotions that accompany the loss of a loved one, I'd like to know about it. One thing I know is that you have to be strong and each day I try to be as courageous as Smokey was.

    Smokey's tombstone reads: "You'll live forever in the hearts of those who loved you."

    Writing this letter has given me the opportunity to talk about Smokey again. I truly cherish these times, even though they hurt.

Most sincerely,

P.P., Missouri

My Dearest Companion

Dear Kymberly,

Your request for people to share with you their stories of losing an animal friend was very timely as just last Thursday, I had to fulfill the terrible responsibility of having my dog euthanized. I am deeply shaken by this and am having problems coping. I know that the memories of a person who is in the throes of grief do not make easy reading, but maybe some of the things I can share in the telling will be of value to those of you who read my story.

    My dog's name was Rocky. He was a huge, black, 160-pound mountain of a Newfoundland — gentle and sensitive, compassionate, intelligent and kind. He came to me through a local Newfoundland rescue organization when he was four years. The people who owned him for his first four years said they couldn't handle his medical problems anymore — he had skin allergies and hip dysplasia. They had confined him to a concrete kennel for most of his life. It isn't hard to imagine the kind of damage that close confinement can cause, particularly to a dog of his size. When Rocky came to me, he was covered with oozing, infected lesions. He was limping, underweight and withdrawn. Yet I saw in his gentle eyes something very special — curiosity, interest and, of all things, humor.

I had decided to get a dog in the first place because of my hearing loss; I did not yet qualify for a hearing dog, but I needed an extra set of ears around to help me be more aware of my environment. When I found out about the animal rescue operation, I contacted them and got Rocky.

Newfs are renowned for their intelligence and power of discernment, their great strength coupled with gentleness and their quiet, whimsical charm, as well as for their sheer hugeness and beauty. Their faces reflect a spirit of benevolence. Rocky had all of these attributes and more. He patiently bore all of the veterinary treatment I foisted upon him. I know he understood that I was only trying to help him.

I did not know at first whether Rocky would bond to me or not, especially after the way he had been treated by other humans. But he seemed to love me immediately. On the first night we were together, after I finished bathing, brushing and feeding him, he began to follow me everywhere. He climbed right up on my bed, looked down at me and curled up as close to me as he could get. So, now I had a warm gentle teddy bear to cuddle with at night. And he wouldn't leave me, either.

I suffer from anxiety and depression, and Rocky helped me through many long nights of fear and kept my loneliness at bay. He listened to me, he watched me as we talked and I was always filled with awe at his ability to understand my feelings and thoughts. He cared.

The only place I did not take Rocky with me

was to work. Actually, I did manage to sneak him in once, much to the surprise and pleasure of my co-workers. In fact, Rocky attracted a lot of attention everywhere we went — concerts in the park, craft fairs and all kinds of other events. He seemed to thoroughly enjoy everything we did together. He made a lovely, soft pillow to lie on while listening to the local symphony outside. Both children and adults found it hard to resist the temptation to pet him. People remarked on his size, his friendliness and even his good manners. He provided me with a bridge for relating to others. This is hard for me and Rocky gave me a way to overcome my shyness and talk to people. No matter how much attention he was getting, though, he never left me alone. At the least sign of distress in my voice or body language, he was immediately at hand.

    Rocky's passion was riding in the car. I absolutely loved that. He sat right next to me on the front seat, watching the world go by. Every now and then, he would touch his soft nose to my cheek or my hair and give me a whiffle and a kiss. I always felt so privileged that I could win the love of this great, gentle being who had been so deeply wronged in his earlier life. One night Rocky proved his love when he stopped me from stepping out in front of an oncoming car. I didn't hear its approach, but Rocky did and he acted quickly, knocking me back toward the curb. He may well have saved my life.

    It pleased me to watch as Rocky's health improved. He gained weight, his skin cleared up and his coat grew in thick and beautiful. The time I spent brushing, clipping, combing and untangling his fur was soothing for me. Caring for him gave me purpose. His condition improved so much that he took to prancing about with me in my living room when I practiced my dance steps.

    Rocky loved churches and shrines. I remember the evening I took him with me to a local shrine; he became very quiet, very serious and just sat, gazing into the little chapel. One woman there was deeply offended when she saw him and said that a house of worship was no place for a dog. Later, when I tried to leave, Rocky kept pulling me back toward the shrine. He acted the same way on many other occasions, trying to pull me into churches of all kinds during our nightly walks. There was something about sacred places that really seemed to appeal to him.

    Rocky expressed to me in many different ways what he was feeling and thinking. He would lay his great head on my knee or my shoulder and just gaze at me, listening intently and reacting with his eyes. Sometimes he would touch me gently with his massive paws. When he wanted to communicate his feelings, he made use of a wide range of woofs, grunts and gestures.

    After a while, I began to notice signs that some of Rocky's health problems might be returning. It became painful for him when I massaged his paws and legs and shoulders. He began to stumble when he walked, first only occasionally and then more frequently. I knew what was coming, but I so hoped that Rocky would have at least another year. It was not to be.

    I am filled with rage because I feel that his first owners robbed him of the best part of his life because of their laziness and neglect. The giant breeds do not have the life spans of other dogs, but Rocky was cheated out of the short life he had. I will never be able to forgive those people for what they did to him.

And so, last Thursday, a friend and I took my beloved friend to my veterinarian. I told the vet that Rocky seemed to be deteriorating and that I had to know if there was anything that could possibly be done for him. The vet said that there was nothing he could do to help Rocky. And so, I asked that we let Rocky be set free. With compassion and gentleness, the vet told me that the decision I had made was an act of love, the last gift I could give to Rocky — freedom from pain and disability. But I was so afraid to let him go.

Years ago, I worked for a while as a veterinary assistant. I saw things in that job that made me swear to myself that I would never force an animal to stay in a life of misery due to my own cowardice or selfishness. Still, a part of me felt that I was murdering my dearest companion. The vet and his assistant were as kind and supportive as they could be. They explained to me what they would do: first, let me say goodbye for as long as I needed to, then they would administer a tranquilizer to relax him and lessen his pain. This would be followed by the final shot, an overdose of barbiturate. Then he would be free.

I held Rocky and told him how much I loved him. I thanked him for his love and care and devoted protection. He looked up at me with his sweet and gentle eyes and he saw me crying. I felt that I was a killer. I felt terrified. What would I do without having him within reach? Where would I go without him?

That night, I took him to the beach, where he loved to be, for one last walk. (I don't know when I will be able to go back to the beach again.) I cried all over him and held him and he licked my tears away. All too soon it was time for me to bring him back to the vet so that what had to be done could be done. When the final shot was ready and I stood up and gazed at him one last time, Rocky looked at me and his eyes seemed to ask, Momma, where are you going, all upset and without me? It was almost more than I could bear.

I know I did what was right, but I don't know how to handle it. It is hard to sleep, because my gentle teddy bear to snuggle with and talk to. I feel utterly alone and bereft. I am I have been trying to cope with my anger at the selfish behavior of the people who failed in their responsibilities to him and so cheated him out of years of his life. Perhaps it is better to feel anger than an engulfing sense of loneliness.

I knew that I had to find another hearing companion even though my grieving process had only just begun. Just days ago another Newfoundland, a puppy named Luie, came into my life. But bless his heart, he can't "replace" Rocky like everyone seems to think. If only it were that simple.

Last night, Luie came to me and gently got into my lap. He lay his head on my shoulder and I dissolved in tears. I know Luie will become a valued and wondrous Newfie friend, but it will take time. Part of moving on with life is accepting the fact that grieving will continue to be a part of your daily activities for a long time to come.

Sincerely,

K.A., Washington

My Buddy and Protector

Dear Kymberly,

I thought you might like to hear about my dog. When I met my husband seven and a half years ago, he introduced me to his other half — Doc, a mutt who had been his faithful companion for more than 13 years. The thing I remember most about Doc was his eyes. They were the most remarkable eyes I have ever seen. He could communicate with his eyes alone.

When I married my husband, Doc became my dog, too. I couldn't have known at the time what a wonderful gift that was. I spent a lot of time at home during those years, and before long Doc and I had formed a strong attachment. He followed me everywhere; I couldn't even go to the bathroom without him. He would lie at my feet whenever I stopped long enough to give him the chance. I can't tell you how many times I fell over him.

When we took in four cats, Doc became a mother to them. I would always find him lying on the floor with one of the cats curled up next to him. Whenever I answered the door, Doc would rush over and place himself between me and the stranger. Who could ask for a more devoted protector? Odd as this may sound, Doc loved going to the vet's. He always wanted to play with the cats and dogs in the waiting room. I could count on some kind of commotion every time we went for a checkup.

As Doc got older, his health began to deteriorate. He developed cataracts and had a very hard time seeing, but his memory of familiar things wasn't dimmed by his failing eyesight. Arthritis soon became another problem. My mother bought him a rug to stand on when he ate so that he would not slip. Jumping onto the bed or the couch was no longer possible, but he still ran to greet me whenever I came in the door.

As the years went on, Doc spent more and more time at the vet's. He had every test imaginable and as a result we spent more on Doc's health care than we did for the three people and the four cats in our household put together. But nothing was too good for our puppy. He was given shots, pills and everything else that might make him feel better. When he lost control of his bodily functions, we got him doggy diapers. Once when I had to go away for three days, Doc refused to eat or drink. He wouldn't even get up to go outside when nature called. When I returned home he seemed to bounce back, but I could not go away without him after that.

By the time he reached the advanced age of 20, Doc had developed both heart and respiratory problems; only his hearing and sense of smell were left intact. He required constant care, but he was our faithful and dear friend.

Shortly after Christmas two years ago, we made the hardest decision we ever had to make. We knew the time had come to put him to sleep. One morning, my husband took Doc to the vet's and came back without him. My daughter and I hoped my husband would walk in with Doc even though we knew he wouldn't. We all sat holding hands, not saying anything for a long time.

For a long time after that, when I came home and didn't see Doc standing there to greet me, I would go looking for him. I even took to creeping around softly at night just in case I might step on him. We still put up Doc's stocking at Christmas even though it's been over a year since he died. Somehow we found it more comforting to leave all of Doc's things just where he had left them. His doggy toys are still on the floor and so are his food and water dish.

I remember worrying about coming home and finding Doc dead, but now I realize that that would have been easier than having to make the decision to end his life. It's true that he had needed a great deal of attention in his last year, but we didn't mind that part. We were willing to spend as much time and money as necessary to make him well and happy. But finally we ran out of options. He was old and dying.

Thank you for taking the time to read my letter. Remembering Doc's antics and how much my family and I gained from having him in our lives has not only kept Doc's memory fresh and bright, but it has also eased our suffering and helped us to carry on.

Sincerely,

R.W., Virginia

My Little Ferret Friend

Dear Kymberly,

Six years ago, having just moved into an apartment, I found myself wanting a pet. I decided on a ferret, primarily because they are small and quiet and they don't require outdoor exercise. I found a six-month-old sable male through a newspaper ad.

    I named him Root Boy — Rudy for short — because he was into *everything*. When I was asleep or not at home, I kept Rudy in his cage where I knew he couldn't get into trouble. However, whenever I was home, he had the run of the apartment. This meant I had to pick up after him continuously. He would pull all the books from the bottom shelf of the bookcase and root around in them, then scamper off, chirping, like he'd really enjoyed himself. He liked to play in paper bags and hide under the furniture, and all I'd see was either his tail or the end of his nose peeking out. If something was light enough for him to carry, he would hide it under the furniture, so when I did laundry I had to look everywhere for my socks and washcloths. Once I walked into the bedroom and saw my tennis shoe banging itself up against the front of my dresser. It took me a minute to realize that it was Rudy under the dresser, furiously trying to pull the shoe in after him!

I found that many people are misinformed about ferrets. They think of them as smelly rodents, wild animals who bite people. Granted, I'm sure there are some that do bite, but not all of them. Rudy was neutered and descented and raised with love and affection and never had a bad attitude.

Late one night last year, Rudy became very ill. I took him to an emergency animal clinic and they diagnosed him as having a form of cancer called lymphosarcoma. The vet suggested that we try chemotherapy even though it is very difficult to administer to ferrets because their veins are so small. And of course there was no guarantee that chemotherapy would do any good. The vet was such a caring doctor and he was so willing to help my friend. His kindness made the decision of whether or not to try the treatment a little easier. I was told that with treatment, Rudy might live for a year, and without it he probably wouldn't live for more than two months. So I decided to send Rudy for the chemotherapy treatment and I gave him his medicine at home every day.

The chemotherapy kept Rudy alive but I noticed that his health was slowly failing. He became weak, tired easily, lost weight and his breathing was sometimes labored. Two months ago, one year after his diagnosis, I took Rudy to the vet for the last time.

All the people there were so kind and compassionate. I will never forget the vet who used to call me to check on Rudy and to offer suggestions. It really meant a lot to me that they cared so much.

    I was able to spend some time with Rudy the day he died and I thought about all the fun I had had with him. Then I said goodbye. I decided to stay in the room while they gave him the shot that ended his life. I didn't want him to think I'd abandoned him and I didn't want him to be frightened. Putting him to sleep was the hardest thing I ever had to do.

    Of course there were people who said, "It's only a ferret," that I shouldn't be so upset, but these people didn't understand. On the other hand, my friends and family and co-workers were sympathetic and seemed able to accept my sadness. They knew that I had been very stressed while Rudy was ill, that I had spent a lot of time (and money) caring for him and that I had made many changes in my work schedule. More importantly, they knew how much I care about my pets, that I consider them part of my family and that I loved Rudy tremendously.

    Euthanasia is never an easy decision. It broke my heart to have to agree to it, but the quality had gone out of Rudy's life. To see a once playful bouncing ball of fur wasting away in front of me was too much to bear. I just couldn't watch him suffer anymore.

    It was hard to tell if Rudy was in pain during his illness because ferrets make very little noise, but sometimes he would whimper in his sleep. When I would drape him across my shoulder, he would snuggle up to my neck — something he could never stay still long enough to do before.

    That last day I cried the entire time I was at the vet's and also the whole way home...with only the empty carrier on the seat next to me. When I think of Rudy it brings tears to my eyes because he was a part of my life for six years and I miss him.

Unfortunately, most pets don't die peacefully in their sleep. And although it may seem a little like playing God, sometimes we have to make the ultimate choice for our dying pets. I know in my heart that I made the right decision. My little friend Rudy isn't suffering anymore.

Sincerely,

S.R., Maryland

A Naturally Centered Being

Dear Kymberly,

My dog Taki was halfway through her tenth year when she died last March. A 35-pound mixed-breed terrier, her main goal in life was to supply me with unending love and devotion. Until the day she died she never lost her puppy-like joy; people were often surprised to hear that she was 10 *years* old and not 10 *months* old. A friend once said that he had never seen any creature more full of love than Taki. He was right.

    I first met Taki when she was eight weeks old and living at an ASPCA in New York City. I had gone to the shelter only to help a friend find a cat and had absolutely no desire to get a dog. But when I walked in and saw this little puppy with her hair sticking straight out, wrestling with and thoroughly frustrating a German shepherd pup three times her size, I simply couldn't resist. I knew right away that this was the dog for me.

    Over time, an emotional and even spiritual bond grew between us. It seemed as if we both knew what the other was thinking and feeling. On those many occasions when my fiancée and I got into a heated discussion, we noticed that Taki would quietly slink away. She didn't like to see or hear us fight. My fiancée (and now my wife) grew to love the dog as much as I did.

Last February we brought Taki to the vet for her semi-annual check-up. We noticed that she had lost two pounds, but I thought this was because we had recently taken her off corticosteroid medication for her allergies.

The vet ran some blood tests and suggested that we might want to have a full set of x-rays done. But because the blood tests came back negative and because Taki was acting normally and showed no signs of illness, the x-rays seemed unnecessary. I was certain the weight loss was due to the medication change.

A few weeks later, we noticed that there was a little discharge following her bowel movements. Because she showed no other signs of illness, we waited until Monday to have her checked out. The vet found a tumor in her pancreas and said immediate surgery was necessary. The night before the operation was the first time Taki showed any signs of being ill. Her stomach became bloated and she refused to eat. That night she slept underneath my side of the bed (not her normal place). I think that maybe she hoped that I would take away her pain, so she stayed near me.

Although I was optimistic that the operation would be successful, I also felt a tremendous sense of powerlessness. During the surgery the vet saw that Taki was riddled with cancer, so much so that she didn't think Taki would recover or even make it through the anesthesia. Even if she did manage to survive the operation, the vet felt strongly that Taki would only live for a few, very painful days. We chose what we believed to be the only humane thing to do and had her put to sleep during the operation.

    The next few days were the most painful of my life. The suddenness of Taki's death left my wife and me completely unprepared. Even my mother's death didn't hit me as hard, but that was perhaps because it was preceded by a long illness which allowed me to be more prepared when she finally died. My wife and I would frequently break into tears (this still happens — I'm crying now as I write this). Taki's death seemed so unfair. I felt as if the center of my soul had been destroyed. Once, when I accidentally moved her old collar, I heard the clang of her dog tags and I thought for one glorious moment that she was still alive. Her absence haunted our apartment. In the days after her death, I was also torn over my previous decision not to get a full set of x-rays. If I only had... she might still be alive.

    During this time, my friends, especially those who had come to love Taki, were very supportive and helped us by talking about the good times we had with her. Some people might find these kinds of memories too painful to talk about, but I believe that it helps to eulogize a pet and to acknowledge how important they were to you.

    I realized that for most of Taki's life I had only been aware of my responsibility to her. I had to feed her, walk her, clean up after her and care for her when she was sick. So many times I couldn't do something or go somewhere because I had to go home and take care of the dog. Of course, I didn't mind this responsibility, but I think it made me blind to all the many things she gave me and to how much I depended upon her.

It was only with Taki's death that I could truly appreciate the companionship and love that she gave me and the truly joyous way she welcomed life. I came to understand that there is a dog's way of living, a sort of canine philosophy, that treats even the most mundane things — like our daily walks — with openness and excitement. No matter what we did, it was okay with her — as long as we did it together. I finally realized that a dog like Taki is a naturally centered being, with a balance that we humans seldom attain.

Three weeks after Taki died, my wife and I started to think about getting another dog to fill the sudden void in our lives. I think that the time we spent grieving for Taki made it possible for us to accept a new dog into our lives so soon after her death without feeling guilty. Within a week we found a wonderful Irish setter puppy. Puppies have this marvelous way of not letting you feel too sad.

I hope my letter will help other people whose pet has just died. I found that it was very helpful to allow myself to experience the grief I felt and to express those feelings fully. There is no need to be ashamed of grieving the loss of a pet and there is certainly nothing to be gained from denying your pain. It doesn't really matter if no one else understands what you are going through. Your grief is real to *you* and only by experiencing it openly can you hope to grow from it. In my case, it also helped a great deal to get another dog once I felt ready to take that step.

Good luck and I hope this letter helps.

D.M., New York

My Little Lu Lu

Dear Kymberly,

My little Lu Lu came into my life several months ago. She was seven weeks old at the time. Although she was an unusually pretty white kitten, my other cat, Emmie, didn't seem to appreciate her lovely qualities. Life was hard for Lu Lu from just about the very beginning. The day after I got her, I took her to the vet for her vaccination and discovered that she also needed to have her ears cleaned of ear mites. As little as she cared for that procedure, she thought even less of having to endure a month of ear mite medication. That was only one of her many early illnesses.

    Luckily, Lu Lu got better and was finally able to experience what it was like to be healthy. Emmie changed her mind about the new family member and the two of them started to play together and soon became great friends. The one thing that endears me to my little Lu Lu is that she was so darn affectionate. She always wanted to be touched and she was especially keen on cuddling when she was going for a cat nap. She would often *insist* that I kiss her by putting her mouth directly on mine.

She was so full of love.

The day came when I moved out of the city to take care of my mother's house in the country while she was away for a few months. I thought this would be great for the cats.

At first, Lu Lu chose to stay around the house. On the second day, I went to work and decided to put her outside so she could explore (she was only three months old at the time and was very curious). When I came home that night, Lu Lu didn't come when I called.

I was filled with a lot of guilt for putting her outside and expecting her to stick around like Emmie does. I rode around on my bike looking for her, knocking on doors and asking people if they'd seen her. I put up signs. But no Lu Lu. I cried for her because I was scared she was out in the big world with no one to love and protect her. Maybe she would become a wild cat and never know a kiss again.

I found that most people don't seem to think that the loss of a pet is very important. Most of the reactions I got were not very compassionate at all. Thankfully, my closest friends, the ones I've always been able to share my true feelings with, have been the best support.

Lu Lu has been missing for two weeks at the time of this letter. Most of the time I try not to think about her because there is nothing I can do. I guess I'm still in the stage they call denial because most of the time I'm still hoping she'll come back.

I feel so sad that it's making me cry to think about this. Even though I only had her for too long, she grew on me very quickly. I love Lu Lu and I miss her. I can only hope she has found a loving home.

When will I stop grieving for her? I wish I knew. People are always asking me when I'm going to get another cat. They don't seem to understand that it isn't a another cat I want, it's Lu Lu. I have to get over her before I can begin to think about another baby.

I would be honored to have you print my letter.

Sincerely,

D.P., Canada

Riding Max's Back

Dear Kymberly,

I am 11 years old. When I was very young, 3 or 4, I had a dachshund named Max. He was old and I was very young but I remember him clearly. He was very friendly toward me and loved to play. We would run around the yard together all of the time. Max was tannish gray. He was also rather protective. I would ride around on his back — that's very hard for dachshunds and I know he didn't like it that much. When he was 13, Max had to be put to sleep. My family said it was because he was suffering and it would be best. Just to think about it used to make me cry. Until about a year ago I thought my riding on his back was the reason he had to be eusianized [sic]. I felt very bad for a long time, but then I found out it was because he had cancer and that made me feel better.

    Although I think about Max a lot, it doesn't hurt as much anymore.

Sincerely,

J.R., Florida

Swept Away

Dear Kymberly,

I saw the notice about your book on the loss of a pet and it could not have been more timely. I have recently joined a therapy group for people who are suffering from post-traumatic stress. You see, the tornado of '89 destroyed everything I ever had including my beloved female cat, Sebastian (Sebbie for short). It has taken me a long time to come to terms with my losses — Sebbie most of all — and it is only recently that I have begun to pick up the pieces. Writing this letter has been a big step forward in my recovery because I have been able to be completely honest and open about my feelings about losing Sebbie. I have never been able to tell anyone, not even the members of my group, just how hard Sebbie's death was for me.

Sebbie was one of the five kittens that our family cat, Ginger, gave birth to. Sebbie was the runt of the litter, a tabby with a face half gray and half orange. We named her Sebastian because at the time we thought she was a male. She was such a sickly kitten that I thought she might have to be put out of her misery and put to sleep. My son begged me to at least give her a chance to get better. Thankfully, I listened to him because Sebbie's health improved completely and she soon became a much-loved member of our family. She grew into a cat that was as sensitive as she was affectionate. She was the sweetest cat I ever knew and we loved her very much.

Some years later, I got divorced and my son and I moved into a two-bedroom apartment with the four cats — Mother Ginger, sisters Sebbie and Patches and a black stray named Midnight. The apartment was small but we got along just fine.

Then came that terrible day, November 15th, when the tornado struck. I left work and made my way home through the rubble in the dark. I couldn't even tell where my apartment building had been. I screamed for my son and I kept calling for my babies. People thought I meant children, but I told them "No, I mean my little cats." I couldn't find any of them.

It wasn't until hours later at the hospital that I was finally reunited with my son. He told me that when the tornado hit, Patches had jumped into his arms, but the force of the winds had ripped her away. I dreaded to think what may have happened to my other cats. I was in shock and numb, but I had to be strong for my son. He had been hurt when a piece of flying debris had ripped into his back and legs, requiring over 50 stitches.

After a sleepless night, I returned to what was left of my home to see what I could salvage. As I looked around, I suddenly noticed that there in the rubble was my Sebbie. She was dead. Her little green eyes were open and the only damage to her body that I could see was a large patch of pink skin on her side where her fur had been torn away. Her body had already grown stiff and she had been dead for several hours. I fell to pieces, just as I am now as I tell you this story...but I *want* to tell you, so I'll go on. I closed Sebbie's eyes and wrapped her in a sheet. I asked my ex-husband to bury Sebbie, but later I discovered that he had just thrown her into a dumpster — he said he didn't know where else to put her. Even though I just nodded my head and didn't say anything, I was very upset and I have always regretted that. Sebbie deserved so much better than to be dumped onto a heap of trash. There would not even be a grave for me to visit, a place to remember her.

    I told my son about Sebbie's death and he cried. I cried too, but again, I had to be strong for him. In the weeks that followed, I cried when I was alone. Over the next several weeks we managed to find our other three kitties. By that time, I had adopted two new cats from the Humane Society and now I had five. There was none that I loved like Sebbie. I was devastated over losing her.

    I finally decided to seek therapy. I found a therapist but she didn't seem to understand that the real source of my pain was the loss of my cat. She kept trying to get me to talk about other things. She thought that grieving for my cat wasn't an important issue.

    Not a single person really knows how I felt about Sebbie but you, Kymberly. A lot of bad things have happened to me over the past two years, but I am now in a support group and am finally getting my life together and I have started to be happy and hopeful for better things in the future. I wish I had known then that there were support groups that help people deal with issues like mine. I have overcome most of the grief I felt for the things I lost in the tornado and I am starting to find some peace of mind over Sebbie's death. Also, putting my thoughts and memories in writing has helped me so much. Thank you for reading my letter and for writing your book.

I was lucky to find Sebbie after the tornado (many of my friends and neighbors never found their pets). It is a horrible thing to wonder if your beloved pet is dead or alive. One of my neighbors is still looking for her kitty. I understand how she feels and it really hurts me when she speaks of her lost cat.

Losing Sebbie the way I did has made me think about my other animals a little differently. I hope that when the time comes for them to pass on, it will be through natural death from old age and not through some disaster or accident. Losing a beloved pet in a disaster has got to be the cruelest blow. I think that even a lingering illness would be better than a sudden accident because it would give me more time to prepare for their passing. Whatever may happen to the remaining members of my family, at least I can say that my experiences have made me stronger and for that I am grateful.

Kymberly, maybe this letter means more to me than it means to you, but I am hoping that something in here will help other people. Thanks again for reading my letter and understanding the pain of my loss.

Initials and home state withheld by request

How Love Can Hurt and Heal

Dear Kymberly,

I read about your project and I want to encourage you because I believe a book on dealing with pet loss could actually save lives. So, I would like to contribute with this letter...

I have always been involved with animals and have always owned one. I even wanted to become a vet, but that never worked out. Looking back, most of the animals I have owned really *needed me* and I think this may be why I experienced so much grief when I lost them. I put their needs before mine; their comfort, health and care were first and foremost. Then there were the animals who chose me; they loved me and displayed a desire to become a part of my life. Either way, I was always there for all of my pets.

My years of being a deputy sheriff caused a lot of damage to my body. Years of smoking, coffee and long night shifts took their toll on me and I ended up with all sorts of health problems. One of the reasons that I am doing so well now is because of my pets. They keep me active, but more important, the love they give me and the love I give them takes care of me in a way that medical science can't.

I want to tell you about two special dogs. They are a good example of what animals can do for you and how they can affect your life. Let's start with my precious Oliver, better known as Ollie. One night, a bulldog breeder in Southern California called me. She said that she had a male English bulldog that she had sold to a couple but when they got divorced they gave the dog back to her. When she got him back her female dogs attacked him and he would not defend himself. She knew how I felt about animals and when she asked me if I wanted him, of course I took him — he *needed* me. When I first saw him, I picked him up — he was several years old at that time — and saw that he was not in good physical shape and that his body was scarred. I brought him home and nursed him back to health. It turned out that he was a real pussycat of a dog.

Ollie was sort of a quiet but goofy dog. His favorite trick was to blow the ashes out of ash trays. He liked to lay on the bottom glass shelf of my two end tables. When he woke up, he would stretch and arch his back; ultimately he broke the top glass of both end tables.

When Ollie was about seven, his kidneys started to fail and he lost control of his bladder. He was quite a mess to care for, but that was okay because I loved him. I told Ollie that I would do my best to take care of him. I started by feeding him prescription dog food. It cost $50 a case, but if he needed it, he would get it. Soon he could not relieve himself, so the vet inserted a catheter into his bladder, but it would always come out. Finally the vet switched the catheter to his penis. I felt sorry for him, but I guess the procedure was needed. After about a week, poor Ollie got a little better. The vet told me that he might live another year but not much more than that. I held Ollie and I told him, "Well, buddy, we'll keep you going for another year."

    The next morning I found Ollie dead. He was lying in a pool of urine. I could not accept that he was gone. The vet had told me and I had assured Ollie that he still had time. And then he had to suffer the ultimate insult — to be found dead in a pool of urine.

    Ollie did not look dead and his body did not become stiff or cold. I spent the next 12 hours holding him and crying. I tried to massage him, breathe into him, talk to him. I felt that I had let him down, that I had lied to him. The worst thing was that I knew that I couldn't help him anymore.

    That night I finally found the strength to dig his grave. I refused to let anyone help me. I wanted this to be my final tribute to Ollie. My wife removed her gold necklace with its cross and put it on him. I made a pillow for his head and covered him so he wouldn't get cold, and then I buried him. Nobody but nobody could really understand how I felt about losing that dog.

    I think Baby is the hardest of my pets to write about. Baby never left me except when I was at work. She snuggled next to me on the bed at night, sat with me in my easy chair and when I was in the bathroom, she would come in and lie on the floor. Several times when I was sick in bed, she would not leave my side to eat or drink for days at a time. We were inseparable.

    As she became older and couldn't get around so well, I carried her up and down the stairs and lifted her off and on the bed and the sofa. I carried her outside to go potty and on occasion, I had to wipe her clean and carry her back into the house. We were never apart.

Everyone knew that Baby was getting older and feared what would happen to me when she finally did pass away. I didn't know myself what would happen. Meanwhile I got sick. I was diagnosed with emphysema and the doctor said I had only one year to live. I did not know who would go first, Baby or me. Most bulldogs only live to the age of seven or eight and she was already thirteen and a half. The vet said the only thing that kept her going was love and that she didn't want to leave me. Both of us were getting sicker and sicker.

Baby started to have spells of losing consciousness. She would suddenly lose control of her bladder and then go into a seizure. It was painful for me to see her gasp for breath and pass out and it was so sad to see her confusion and fear when she came to. I tried to control the seizures with artificial respiration, but it didn't help much. She was so sick, so very, very sick.

When I brought her back to the vet, he discovered that Baby had tumors in her throat and in her stomach. She was in obvious pain. She passed out again during the visit and the vet revived her. He then asked what he could do for me — or rather, what I wanted him to do. I made the decision that the kindest thing to do was to let Baby go. I rushed out and let my wife take care of the arrangements.

Afterward we brought her home. A friend of mine dug a grave in our orchard. This time I could not dig it myself. Instead, I held her and petted her little curled tail until it was time for my friend to take her from me for the last time. Even though it can be painful, I think it's important for people to see and feel the dead body of their pet because this makes it easier to accept the reality of the loss — at least it did for me.

Shortly after that, I took a turn for the worse and became sicker and weaker by the day. In retrospect, I can honestly say that I did not want to die, but I didn't really care if I did.

Then one rainy day, my son brought me the most wonderful letter I have ever received. It was from a complete stranger — a nurse in San Francisco. She said that she was so sorry when she heard that I had lost Baby. She expressed sympathy and said a lot of nice things. Then she ended the letter by saying that she hoped I would start taking better care of myself. What a shock! This stranger understood. I had cried when Baby left and I cried when we buried her, but the tears that I shed when I read that letter were for a different reason. That there was another person who understood my grief made such a huge impact on me; it felt like a huge weight had been lifted from my shoulders. With that, I got out of bed, got dressed and I soon started to feel better. That was almost two years ago and I have been feeling better ever since. All of the other pets in our household have made an effort to spend time with me. We all needed each other and although they weren't Baby, that they were there for me meant a lot.

I believe in God, but I am not a religious person. I do know without a doubt that God loves animals, and I figure that because he put them on earth, he must want them to be taken care of. He watches over them and he knows what happens to them. Remember the verse in the Bible about God knowing when even a sparrow falls?

I do not believe that animals are just like humans, but I know that they have the same feelings and emotions. They get hot and cold and feel pain and anguish. They like praise and don't like getting scolded. They show fear and courage. I don't think that animals are human, but I am often reminded that humans are animals.

While some people grieve terribly when they lose a pet friend, others really don't seem to care at all. There are some who only feel bad until they replace the pet and there are others who may not be able to eat for a day or two. For those of us whose pets are our true companions, whose pets take the place of a human loved one, losing them can be completely devastating.

I call all of my dogs "my kids." Of course, I don't really consider them my children, but in an odd way, they take the place that my children used to occupy. I give them the time and attention that I used to give to my children.

I have a few suggestions for people who have lost a beloved animal friend. Make an effort to accept the fact that your pet is dead. One thing that helped me was to actually see and look at the dead body. Yes, it hurt, but it helped me accept the fact that the animal *was gone*. Also, realize that *it is okay* to feel and express your grief. How can you get through the loss if you suppress your feelings? Another thing is that many, many people feel the same way you do; you are not alone and you are not foolish, stupid or crazy for feeling the way you do. There *are* people out there who care.

Of course, there are people who are cold-hearted about these things, who make fun of you because they think it's ridiculous to feel such pain over the loss of an animal, but I believe there are more people who don't feel this way. And anyway, who cares what others think? If all the people who grieve for their pets were to come out of the closet, it would help those of us who are afraid to express our true feelings, afraid of ridicule and afraid that other people won't understand.

My grief almost killed me and I don't want others to have to suffer like I did. It is for this reason that I have written this letter about my grief and my feelings for animals and opened up to you more than I ever have to anyone else in the world. I hope it will help at least someone...

Best wishes,

W.T., California

Tribute to a Gray Furry Friend

Dear Kymberly,

Scooter was a very small bundle of gray fur when she was found by my daughter inside a box in the parking lot of a shopping mall. The family could not resist a bunny who was so cute and cuddly, and a special place was created for her in my daughter's bedroom. Every morning as my daughter dressed for school, Scooter would romp on her bed to lift her spirits. The rest of the day she spent running around the house, taking the stairs at a bound and playing with anyone who happened to have the time and inclination. Scooter was trained to use a litter box and would wait patiently in the laundry room until someone let her out into the garage where the box was kept. When no one was available for play, she would lie in the living room, directly in front of the TV, whether it was turned on or not.

    With each new day, Scooter became more like a member of the family. She had her meals along with everyone else and even went along on family vacations and trips to the store. She was given treats of all kinds, but her favorites were chocolate chip cookies, ice cream and crackers. She also became a kind of good luck mascot at my son's baseball games.

The years passed and my daughter became engaged. Although at first her fiancé insisted that Scooter could not live with them when they got married, that is exactly what happened. She settled into their new home and was given every kind of toy and rabbit-style comfort imaginable. Later she was joined by a puppy and two baby bunnies. She did not think much of the new arrivals and would stomp her back feet in annoyance when they were near.

Scooter loved to come to my house to play in the big yard and lie under her favorite bush. She also had a favorite rug that only she was permitted to sit on. At Christmas, Scooter was given many gifts, ranging from cookies and toys to her own private tent for sleeping in and a car bed for traveling. Some people thought that my daughter and her husband were being silly to dote so on a rabbit, but they didn't know of the joy that Scooter gave them. Whenever Scooter got sick, they would drop everything and rush her to the vet. They could not bear to see her suffer or be in any kind of pain.

When Scooter got sick for what turned out to be the last time, they tried everything to make her well again. When they realized that there was nothing more they could try, my daughter and her husband made the hard decision to end her suffering in a kind and gentle way. They took her to the vet together and stayed with her as she slipped into a peaceful and pain-free sleep.

It is a comfort to think that Scooter was treated in death as she was in life, with the utmost care and love. She was laid to rest in her own beautiful coffin on the grounds of a well-kept cemetery with other beloved pets. Her grave marker bears a rose and her name along with a holder for cut flowers. Visiting Scooter in this lovely place has given us an opportunity to put aside our other concerns and give our thoughts only to her. We have learned that burying your pet in a pet cemetery can be very helpful. It allows you to maintain a relationship with your departed animal. It also helps us to give tribute to our smallest family member and to think back on the wonderful times we shared.

Sincerely,

G.L., Pennsylvania

Animals Are Better

Dear Kymberly,

I remember the first time I set eyes on my kitten, Magic. I happened to notice him at the local pound while I was searching for my missing cat, Panthera. I didn't choose Magic because he had attractive black and white fur. I chose him because he climbed up the side of the cage to greet me.

I took him with me on my first day of school at the California Institute of the Arts and he slept in my lap during orientation. Magic loved to spend his days with me in class sitting on the desk. The teacher loved him and the other students did too. Everyone wanted him to stay on their desk. Not surprisingly, he was a big attraction in the animation department.

Magic saw me through a number of difficult experiences in the years following school. He stayed by me through my divorce and through a period of drug dependency and homelessness.

As soon as my life was on the mend, Magic developed a hacking cough. My boyfriend thought he might have asthma. One day after work we took him to the vet. The vet listened to him and told us to go get something to eat while he ran some tests.

When we came back, I heard Magic cry out and I knew something was wrong, but my boyfriend said I was being paranoid, that everything was probably fine. We were called into the examination room. The vet told us that Magic had feline infectious peritonitis and that it was deadly. He said he could try drugs but that the chances of survival were not good. Also, because Magic was infectious, I had to consider the health of my other cats.

I was faced with the awful decision of whether or not Magic should be put to sleep. Worse yet, I had no time to think about it. I knew that I didn't want Magic to suffer and I didn't want my other cats to be infected. The only logical decision, it seemed, was euthanasia.

First they shaved Magic's leg. The shaving scared him and that upset me. Then the vet injected the needle and he became limp in my arms. I cried more than I have at any time in my life — even more than after the accidental death of my boyfriend.

I went back to my parents' house. They asked what was wrong and when they found out, their only response was an indifferent "I'm sorry." When I continued to cry that day, they told me to snap out of it. When my depression lasted more than two days, they told me to act like a "real person" again. How could I? Magic was my best friend. Two days wasn't enough time to grieve. Two years has not been long enough. My dad told me I was acting silly. Later, he found out what it felt like when the family dog had to be put to sleep after 19 years of life. It was the first time I'd ever seen him cry.

No one was there for me when Magic died.

No one even believed that being there for me was the decent thing to do. How can anyone think that just because Magic was an animal, his death is any less worthy of grieving than a human's?

I often find myself thinking that animals are better than people. They are there for you when humans let you down. They don't care who you are. And they love you regardless of what you do.

A.G., *California*

My Closest and Best Friend

Dear Kymberly,

I am 15 years old. Last May, I lost my closest and best friend and I would like to tell you my story.

When I was six, my mother took me to a nice woman's house where I met two puppies, brother and sister. I chose the female and named the adorable golden retriever Blondie.

I grew up with Blondie and taught her many things. She was loyal, humorous and very loving. I remember once my father forgot to put some steak away. He left it on a coffee table no more than a foot tall. In the morning, it was still there. Blondie loved steak and she could easily have taken it.

When my parents got divorced when I was 10 or 11, I would get upset and cry quietly so my mother wouldn't hear me. Blondie, usually watching TV with my mom, would come back and tried her best to make me smile. Once I forgot to set my alarm for school, but I woke up on time because a dog was staring me hard in the face. She knew I had to wake up, and she also wanted to play.

I shared my deepest thoughts with her and she always listened. I realize now that it wasn't just a one-way street and that she taught me very valuable things about life, too. She taught me faith, loyalty and trust.

Last spring, Blondie decided to chase an animal out of our yard; suddenly, she screamed painfully. I was scared to death that she was hurt and when I couldn't get her to move, I ran screaming to Mom who brought her into the house. When we took her to the vet, we found out that Blondie had broken her front left leg at the shoulder. It was weakened by bone cancer. The vet said her leg had to be amputated, but I refused to let Blondie go through chemotherapy because I knew she didn't need to throw up all the time. The doctor said that she wouldn't live more than three to six months. But he was wrong. Blondie was so wonderful! She returned to her old self and outlived the vet's forecast.

A year later, Blondie got really sick and it went on for weeks. She was vomiting and she was so weak that she couldn't walk by herself. I brushed her every day and prayed she would get better.

The last night I was with Blondie I didn't know it would be the last, but I cried for hours because I knew that she was in so much pain. The next day she went to the vet's and she had to stay overnight. That night she died in her sleep. The next day was my dad's birthday. We buried her next to a dog I had never known, but my parents had him before me. My family let out feelings that I had never seen before and my friends were very supportive, but even today I am mourning. She was the best thing in my life.

My grades this year are much lower and I don't like the way I am. Blondie was so beautiful and so intelligent. There is no one in the world,

human or animal, that I would ever love more.
    Thank you for listening to my emotional tale. No one will ever know what Blondie was like and I can't explain it, but I could die sometimes, I just miss her so much.

Sincerely,

J.S., Pennsylvania

Love of the Wild

Dear Kymberly,

His name was The Gypsy Margay and, obviously, he was a margay, a wild cat found in Central and South America. Also known as long-tailed cats, margays are similar in their markings to an ocelot. They have become rare in much of their native habitat due to unregulated hunting for their valuable fur and kidnappings to meet the growing demands of the exotic pet trade.

    Gypsy came to live with me in the spring of 1968, while my husband was in Vietnam. He had been smuggled out of South America, only to be placed in quarantine by the state of Louisiana, and eventually became an unlikely new addition to the menagerie of animals for sale in a Shreveport pet store. When I came upon Gypsy, he was about six months old — scared and looking mistreated and sick. Unable to simply pass him by, I decided to give Gypsy a real home. With the help of a zoologist friend and because I had a basic understanding of cats, I was able to make surprising progress. In time Gypsy became my confidant, my protector and best friend (next to my husband) and all-around good fellow.

We became inseparable. Gypsy slept with me, played with me, and comforted me when I was sick. He read my moods like most people read a book, and he protected me from anyone who raised his suspicions. In many ways, Gypsy was as devoted as a dog, but his was not a blind devotion. His respect and trust had to be earned. People who owned more conventional pets were puzzled by him or afraid of him; they just didn't understand how a wild jungle cat could be so much a part of the fam-ily. I even encountered a few people who thought he should be mounted on a wall like some sort of trophy.

As the years went by, Gypsy remained happy and active, but my husband and I began to detect some of the usual problems associated with advancing age. We sometimes thought about what we would do when "the time" came, but it was easier not to think about it. Easier, that is, until the gradual failure of his internal organs became a reality. One day I came home from work and found Gypsy bleeding from his nose, ears and rectum. I rushed him to the vet, but he did not recover. After 16 years of friendship, there was nothing more I could do for Gypsy except to give him what has now become known as a "good death."

My first reaction was total irrational anger at my husband, who certainly didn't deserve it. I didn't even call him at work and tell him what happened. I even let him look for Gypsy when he came home and when he asked me where Gypsy was, all I said was "he's dead." That's all I would say about it. My husband was mystified by my behavior. I wouldn't tell him what had happened or why Gypsy was dead. I wouldn't even talk to him. Of course it wasn't my husband's fault, but that's how my grief showed itself at first. When I returned home I cleaned up the blood, threw away all of Gypsy's toys and things, and kept quiet. I had nothing to say. To anyone. I didn't cry. My poor husband had no idea what was going on with me. I just went on as if Gypsy had never existed. I figured that if there had never been a Gypsy, then his death had never happened and I couldn't be hurt or sad. And if there had never been a Gypsy, there was no need to cry.

My husband told our neighbors and friends what had happened and told them not to bring up the subject of Gypsy's death when talking to me. For my part, I never made any mention of the subject at all. Things continued like this for a couple of weeks.

Then one day I found one of Gypsy's favorite toys under the sink in the bathroom. The world crashed in on me and I finally broke down. The tears that I had denied myself flooded from my soul.

Seeing that I was grieving openly, my friends abandoned their silence and tried to find the right words to comfort me, but it only made things worse. They said things like:

"I'm sorry. I don't know what to say. He was nice."

"I guess you don't realize your pets are not immortal until something like this happens. You just figure they will be with you forever."

Others had far less diplomatic things to say:

"Oh grow up! He was just a cat for God's sake."

"He wasn't the sort of cat you should have as

a pet. Most people shoot cats like that and mount them on the wall."

Others tried a little humor:

"Well, at least now I can come over without being afraid that that wild thing would eat me."

Well, the years have passed, I don't cry anymore (getting misty-eyed writing this letter), but there is a deep spot inside me that can never be filled. And near that spot is a place full of memories that is guarded by the thought that I am much better off for having owned (correction — no one ever owns a cat), or rather for having known and loved Gypsy. Whenever I am down or stressed out, I just remember my friend.

I've learned some valuable things while struggling through my grief. One of them is that having people around who don't know what to say is sometimes worse than being alone with your painful thoughts. Also, that if you become terribly attached to an animal friend, one day you will lose him. But for me, pets are part of what makes life worth living, so even though a loss like this can be so devastating, it's worth it. Another thing I've learned is that reading about the experiences of others who have lost a beloved pet can help you understand that you are not alone and that your feelings, however strong or strange they may be, are a normal part of letting go.

Sincerely,

E.G., California

Separation Blues

Dear Kymberly,

I have had pets for as long as I can remember, and I am no stranger to the loss of these companions, but nothing ever affected me like the loss of my German shepherd mix, Bambi.

    Some time after my parents split up in a bitter divorce, my father and his new wife asked me to come and live with them. It was my first year of high school and they told me that my mother wasn't caring for me as well as she could. They promised me that I would have a real family where there was dinner on the table every night and security and consistency — things I never had, even when my family was together. Even though I was intrigued by the idea of having a more stable family life, of finally having my own room, of being the only child living in the house and getting away from my two sisters who I didn't get along with, I was still unsure. The deal was cinched when my father said I could have a dog.

    I had a dog, but because I was a little terror, the dog avoided me, preferring the company of my older sisters. I moved in with my father, looking forward to the new and wonderful life that lay ahead of me.

Several months after I settled down as a freshman in high school, I decided it was time to cash in on his promise. With a little hesitation on my father's part, we headed to the local Animal League and looked at dogs. Even though I would have liked a puppy, I knew I didn't have the time to train one.

I didn't choose Bambi — my father did. He said she was the only dog who didn't whine and jump in her cage. She had pride and she stood stoically in her cage, even though she was desperate to get out of it.

From the day she came home with us, she knew she belonged to me. She trusted me and I trusted her. For example, even though we lived in the city, she never needed a leash. The level of communication between us was amazing.

My father and I went through some really rough times and I had many problems with my mother as well. I guess I was going through the tribulations that troubled teens are prone to during high school. As I struggled through this hard period, Bambi was my rock. She was the best dog I ever could have asked for. Even though friends of mine often commented that Bambi was very mellow — too mellow for them — she was perfect for me. When my father and his wife began spending weekends at their new home that they were going to live in when I went to college, Bambi became an especially valued friend.

Right after I learned that I was accepted at a college in upstate New York, I was informed that Bambi could not stay with my father. He said that he would not keep the dog until I was able to settle down somewhere. From then on, all I did was dread the near future.

    I was offered a three-week trip to Florida the summer after my junior year. My mother said she would take Bambi while I was gone. I didn't have as good a time as I had hoped. About halfway through my vacation, while speaking to my mother, she commented on how the next-door neighbors had taken to Bambi, especially their little girl. A few days later, my parents told me that because Bambi had to be given away soon, they had decided to give her to the neighbors. At least I could visit her, they said. When I objected, I was told that taking Bambi away from our neighbors' little girl would devastate her. I was the one who was devastated.

    The loss of Bambi affected my life so greatly that I could hardly function. The pain in my heart was so great that I sank into a major depression that has taken years of therapy to deal with. When they took away the only thing I loved, it brought back all the issues of my troubled childhood.

    When I visited Bambi, it was hard on the little girl because Bambi wanted to be with me and not her. Everyone around me thought I was overly dramatic. Nobody could understand this kind of attachment to a dog. It took me six years to find a friend who could understand the pain I was experiencing.

    After Bambi was gone, everyone kept reminding me how lucky I was to know that my dog had gone to a good home where she would be loved. It was almost as if my own love for her wasn't enough. The most ironic thing was that less than two years later, after I had dropped out of college, I settled in a place where I could have brought

Bambi to live.

    I guess it was too much to ask my family — rather, the people who were supposed to be my family — to take care of her for me. Bambi was more "family" to me than any human has ever been. I still feel angry about it and as I write this letter I'm crying.

    Two years ago I adopted a rambunctious puppy I call Roxie. She lives with me and my fiancé. We went through some pretty tough times with her during her training. She was aggressive and difficult. There were points when my fiancé told me to get rid of her, but there is no way I will ever let a person come between me and my dog again.

Sincerely,

J.H., New York

"Mom, Gussie Died"

Dear Kymberly,

Sometimes I find it hard to believe that I had a cat for 21 years. But she was not just any cat — she was a Siamese. And as anyone who has ever lived with a Siamese cat will quickly agree, they are a wonderful breed.

    Her name was Gussie — an unusual name for a breed that usually gets a more exotic title. Gussie was only six weeks old when my son got her. He took care of her for a while, but when he became a teenager, he gradually lost interest in his pet and before I realized what was happening, I found myself taking care of her. It was the first time I had ever had an up close and personal relationship with a Siamese and she lived longer than any cat I had ever known.

    One weekend I had to be away from home and away from Gussie. When I returned, I thought it was strange that there were no friendly cat meows to greet me. My daughter must have sensed my worry because rather than asking me about my trip or saying she was glad to see me, she looked straight at me and said quietly and simply, "Mom,

Gussie died." At first I had no words to offer in reply. When at last I found them, I could only repeat the usual expressions of disbelief. After more than 20 years it was nearly impossible for me to accept the fact that my Gussie was gone.

For months I went about my daily activities, but I was a changed person. Hard as it must be for those who have never had a longtime animal friend to grasp, I would actually catch myself looking for Gussie, especially first thing in the morning, at mealtimes and in the evening. Then it would hit me, and I can't describe the letdown that never failed to engulf my whole being — I wasn't going to find Gussie — not that day or ever again. I even dream about that cat — her special walk, her slightly crossed blue eyes, how she would manage to look me straight in the eye for what seemed like hours without blinking or moving her head.

The events I've been talking about took place more than 20 years ago, but even today as I think back and picture my special friend Gussie, I still get a lump in my throat.

Yours truly,

P.G., Oregon

Bestest House Mouse Ever

Dear Kymberly,

Until this past spring I had an unusual pet named Spot — a white mouse with black spots (hence his *unusual* name!). Because Spot was more than two years old at the time of his death, I assumed that he died from simple old age. But perhaps I should start at the beginning...

    I bought Spot as a very juvenile mouse from a new litter at a pet store. I *never* picked him up by his tail and instead taught him to jump on my hand when I wanted to pick him up. I also trained him never to bite by lightly flicking his nose with my thumb and forefinger when he did.

    I gave Spot occasional free run of my bathroom (but only after shoving a blanket under the door to fill in the space). I couldn't give him free run of the apartment because of my roommate's revulsion and because there were many gaps in the woodwork going who knew where. So I spent a lot of time playing with him on the bathroom floor.

    When I moved to a new apartment with a new roomie (who also happened to be my boyfriend), Spot had free run of the place — but only while we were home and only during the day. He was now an adult and a mousy little mouse, but he was definitely people-oriented. When I'd walk into a room and stop, Spot would run up to me. If I didn't pick him up, he'd attempt to climb up my leg — very ticklish if I wasn't in jeans! He would run into the kitchen whenever anyone went in there. Even in his little mouse-brain, he knew the kitchen meant food! It got to the point where Spot would have to be put in his cage during dinner because he would beg so much.

No one, not even my boyfriend, could quite figure out how I could love a mouse so much. But Spot was so tiny and defenseless and completely trusting of me, how could I *not* love him? His antics and sometimes even acrobatics could keep me amused for hours. I even tried to figure out a way to make a small harness and leash so he could go outside in the summer for walks. That never did work out, though.

Spot was now in his mousy prime. He had plenty of exercise, plenty of things to climb and crawl through or behind for healthy curiosity and lots of "Spotcrumbs" (little crumbs of bread, cereal or cake that we used as rewards).

Then we moved again. This new apartment had too many gaps and holes, so Spot could no longer have the free run he had grown used to. We got him an exercise ball and he was both pathetic and hilarious to watch as he tried to learn to move and navigate by new rules. He did it, however, and quite well. He could speed up to go over the door frame and stop on a — well, a quarter. Darn good for a mouse!

When Spot came down with a case of the sniffles, I filled the bathtub to the rim with steaming hot water, put Spot's cage beside it and turned on the small electric heater. Then I shut the door and kept him in there for a few hours to ease his horrible congestion. I also gave him raisins and raisin bran cereal and Fruit Loops (for vitamin C because he would *not* lick up orange juice). All this usually worked.

After about a year or so, Spot started slowing down. Sometimes he didn't come out of his cage more than once or twice a week. I started letting him run on the kitchen table, with an old blanket thrown on it, making mouse-sized tunnels and caves, or on the bed, to stimulate his curiosity and give him some exercise. It seemed to work for a few months, but then we moved again. Once we finally got settled in, Spotmouse didn't respond to any "remedy" I could think of. He wouldn't roll in his ball — he'd just sit in it. He would merely curl up in a blanket and sleep on the bed. One afternoon, I found him dead in his cage. He wasn't even cold or stiff yet.

I called my boyfriend at work and he came rushing home for me. I'd been saying for months now that when Spotmouse died, I'd need a week off work, so I guess he understood — finally — how much I loved Spot.

Waiting for him to come home, crying my eyes out, I made a tombstone out of a cassette tape cover with his name, approximate birthdate and death date and my favorite Spotmouse saying — "The bestest housemouse ever." Then I wrapped him in a piece of satin and we buried him between the bushes in front of the porch.

For days, I'd sit out on the porch and look at his tombstone. It would make me remember some silly little mousy thing he'd done and even though

I'd cry, it would make me feel better. My family and friends, however, were less than overly sympathetic. When told the news, some said "Oh," some "Sorry," and most made no reply at all. After all, they must have thought, how could anyone love a *mouse*?

Fortunately, I do have a few pictures of Spot and one of them is going in my collage of family photos.

I couldn't clean out his cage for the final time, so I made my boyfriend do that. Until recently, even though I'd watch the mice at pet shops, I didn't want another. Now I'm thinking maybe after Christmas I'll get another mouse, or maybe a puppy. I'll see.

I hope my letter, much longer than I had intended, will help the people who read your book. Owners of unconventional pets need to know that their grief is every bit as real as owners of other types of animals and the lack of sympathy that others may show (even cat and dog owners) is not right. My advice? Ignore those who don't seem to care and seek solace in your own memories.

Sincerely,

M.G., Ohio

The Scales of Memory

Dear Kymberly,

It was during my second trip to Mexico that I was invited to the home of an elderly anthropologist and his wife. He promised me that our dinner would include a very special dish, one he was reasonably sure I hadn't tried before.

    On the appointed night I was ushered onto a patio and offered a selection of savory appetizers to accompany our tequila cocktails. We talked amiably until at last a bell was sounded for dinner. I was seated at the head of the dining table. Not far from me was a large covered serving tray; it remained covered until our wine glasses were filled and various side dishes were passed around the table. Then with a flourish, my host removed the domed cover to reveal one of the most beautifully presented entrees I had ever seen. I mistook the succulent chunks of meat for lean but wonderfully seasoned pork. My host allowed me to continue to think this until the platter was nearly emptied of its delicious contents. It was then that I discovered that what I had been eating with such unconcealed relish was a slow-cooked ragout of mountain

iguana. I had been spending the last hour savoring mouthfuls of lizard — and giant lizard at that.
I must admit that the experience gave me a new respect for a creature long a part of the Mexican landscape. I decided to read up on the scaly beast, and I learned that it was considered both a delicacy and an excellent pet by many generations of Indians. Capable of growing to more than five feet in length, the iguana was renowned for its gentleness as well as its sometimes fearsome appearance. Considered a resourceful hunter and a guardian animal with courage that could rival most dogs, this much-maligned lizard was a lot more complex than I'd ever suspected.

    I suppose that I shouldn't have been surprised when, about two years later, an opportunity to get to know an iguana on more intimate terms presented itself. A friend who had suffered through my overdone descriptions of my Mexican feast offered me a most unusual challenge: Would I be willing to adopt a young iguana who was in need of a home? Remembering that I still had a 75-gallon terrarium in my basement, I jumped at the chance. My friend made me promise never to even think about dropping this innocent creature into a boiling stew pot or onto a blazing grill.

    After being introduced to Armando, the thought of making a recipe out of him was the farthest thing from my mind. He took to the terrarium almost instantly and transformed its arid space into a very personalized lair. The high point of our days became mealtime when Armando would walk up my arm to retrieve large, juicy beetles from my shoulder. He became quite adept at finding cleverly concealed insect morsels around the house, and before long I gave up trying to outwit him.

When another friend appeared one day with an elaborate, handmade leash, I thanked her but expressed serious doubts that Armando would allow such a device to be strapped around him. My friend insisted that there would be no harm in giving the leash a try, and I reluctantly consented. To my utter amazement, Armando made no fuss at all and almost seemed to be assisting me with the curious contraption. I was prepared to begin dragging him toward the door when he strode bravely to the threshold, impatiently pulling on the lead for me to follow. The sight of a three and a half foot lizard promenading along the sidewalk, his head held high, with his human "owner" in tow made more than a few neighbors stop dead in their tracks. Two rather large and usually surly cats took one look at Armando and bolted across the street and into a low-hanging tree.

Although he often had to be bribed with a few especially tasty insect treats, Armando could be persuaded to perform for guests. His performances often consisted of removing shoes and sometimes even socks from unsuspecting visitors, but once he leapt from one chair to another, landing perfectly between a woman's outstretched arms.

Life with Armando continued to be a constant delight until one day I noticed that he had grown peculiarly listless. By early evening, he seemed to be clutching his underside. Alarmed by his unusual behavior, I contacted an acquaintance who specialized in writing feature articles about "exotic animals." He was able to refer me to a retired zoo curator with his own custom-designed examination room in his basement. Armando was almost immobile by the time I got him to the makeshift clinic. I waited outside at the insistence of the elderly curator; he hinted that examinations involving a stomach probe were not a pretty sight.

To make a painful story mercifully shorter, Armando did not survive his examination. He had somehow ingested a collapsible kitchen whisk a few days earlier, and the vicious implement had played havoc with his internal organs. By the time he was brought for treatment it was already too late.

I knew that the only way I could deal with this sudden loss was by giving Armando a funeral worthy of his special place in my heart. I contacted one of my co-workers whose hobby was tackling the more challenging aspects of cabinet-making. We discussed my idea of commissioning a special, one-of-a-kind casket to hold my beloved iguana. After researching the matter at our local university library, my very obliging friend presented me with a measured drawing of a beautiful oblong case bearing authentic Aztec friezework. We settled on a price for labor and materials and within a week the casket was completed. It was far more impressive than the working drawing foretold, and I was moved nearly to tears.

My old friend, the Mexican anthropologist, and his wife actually flew up for the obsequies; I was genuinely touched that the person who had introduced me to the wonders of the fabled iguana would care enough to be present. Nearly two dozen friends and acquaintances attended the viewing and subsequent interment. During the burial ceremony, a few uninvited onlookers were heard to make some uncalled-for remarks about the occasion, but most of the people who came were pleased to be able to take part in a truly unique commemoration. A reporter from the local newspaper arrived with the intention of writing a satirical feature piece but came away with a very different idea. He had seen through the surface oddity of the ceremony and recognized a larger truth: When people are grieving the loss of an animal companion, whether it's a dog or cat or a very large lizard, the honor they give to the memory of that departed creature can be a salve for the soul.

I very much doubt that I will replace Armando with another of his kind (and I certainly wouldn't dream of dining on any of his myriad relations), but I will find solace in the sheer delight of the times we spent together.

B.F., Pennsylvania

A Lady and a Fat Rabbit

Dear Kymberly,

I am writing to share with you the joy and the loss of two very dear friends. It has been a little over two years since my dog and my rabbit died within 11 days of each other. Today they are buried side by side beneath the fir tree in my back yard.

My Red Dog was a beautiful, intelligent field Irish setter, and very much a lady. We shared each other's company for 13 years. I met Red Dog when she appeared one day at the little house I had rented with a group of friends in one corner of a large farm. Some time afterward, I happened to meet her owner. When he said he wanted to get rid of his dog, I told him I was interested. When I went to pick her up, I told her she was welcome to come with me if she wished. Without a moment's hesitation she jumped into the front seat of my car and thus began our life together.

Red Dog could swim across the Kentucky River and chase rabbits all day, go anywhere unleashed and have perfect manners. She watched over my two children, she saved my husband and I from being mugged one night on a beach, she prevented an attack by a growling pit bull on me and my three-year-old son, and she let two threatening farm dogs know that they were not to harm me. She was a very special lady.

In the last year of her life, Red Dog aged quickly. We still enjoyed our daily walks in the rolling fields, but her pace had become much slower. When Red Dog became incontinent, I could sense that she was embarrassed and felt degraded. She began to act so oddly, sleeping all day and whining and pacing and panting endlessly throughout the night. We tried everything we could think of to ease the anxieties that tormented her when the sun went down. Once the sun came up, she was okay again. What was happening to her at night was a mystery to us. It was so sad. Something was wrong, somewhere she was in pain but I didn't know where.

After talking to the vet, my husband and I realized that we had to put her to sleep. My vet did it in the back of my station wagon. I will never forget Red Dog on her final day — she looked so beautiful and dignified as she watched the vet prepare for the injection. Then her beautiful head dropped and she was gone. I cried for a long time afterwards.

My husband was wonderful about helping me. He and a friend buried Red Dog for me. They dug a grave beneath the fir tree in our yard. My family, my friends and the people at work were all very kind and understanding.

For years, whenever I would go somewhere, I would think to myself, "Oh, I have to go get Red Dog." It was a momentary lapse of memory — I would forget that she was no longer here — even after so much time had gone by.

After a year had gone by, I decided that I was ready to get another dog, but I wanted to find one of a different breed. I've known people who believe that choosing a dog of the same breed as the one they've lost will make it easier to overcome their pain. I know that if it is done to try to find a replacement pet with the same personality as the one who died, the effort is bound to fail. Also, it is sad for the new dog. True dog people know that personalities are not interchangeable and they will cherish their new pet for all her unique qualities without forgetting their departed friend. So, I got a new buddy — a 112-pound Akita puppy named Bear. My family took to him immediately and he has kept us busy in all sorts of weather, roaming over hill and dale and having fun in places most sane dogs and people wouldn't dream of going. It pleases me to think that if Red Dog had met Bear, he would have liked him.

It's time for me to introduce the other main character in this story. My husband had stopped by a local pub sometime during the last year of Red Dog's life. He was surprised to find, sitting on the bar, a large gray and white rabbit whose long ears stood straight up. The owner agreed to part with the frightened creature, and my husband brought him home as a gift for my daughter. Once he had taught himself to use a litter box, Thumper was given the run of the house (we hate cages). Late each afternoon, we turned him loose in our fenced-in back yard. After a few hours, we'd bring him in for the night. Well, catching a rabbit in a big yard was comical and extremely difficult, so I gave up trying. It only frightened him, so we let him be and spoke kindly to him whenever we went outside — which was all the time since it was June. The children were not allowed to chase him — we were *developing trust,* we told them. He had plenty of good things to eat, he leveled my garden to dust and took naps under the big holly tree. I would bring his bowl of pellets out into the yard and rattle the bowl while calling his name. Soon he started coming a little closer each day.

Like most Irish setters, Red Dog's passion was chasing wild rabbits. When Thumper came to live with us, we told Red Dog to leave him alone and that's all we ever had to say about it again. It turned out that Thumper loved to follow Red Dog about and lie down next to her on the back porch, and even hopping back and forth over her while she was napping. Thumper was a real character.

One summer day there was a freak thunderstorm. After getting the children and Red Dog into the dry kitchen, I brought in the two soggy cats. I saw Thumper hiding under a bush getting soaked and I simply walked over, picked him up gently and brought him into the kitchen. What a group! The children, the cats, old Red Dog and one fat wet rabbit! It was fun — we stayed together, all of us listening to the storm and snacking on goodies in the kitchen. After that day, Thumper began to come into the kitchen for brief visits and in time he would scratch at the back door whenever he wanted to come in or out.

Thumper and I became very close. He would even meet me at the back gate with Red Dog when I returned home from working the night shift at the hospital. I'd sit on the back step and drink a cup of coffee and Thumper would let me stroke his long transparent ears. He would leap three feet in the air and kick wildly about or twist and run madly about — just for the fun of it. He was so comical to watch, he always made me smile. He enjoyed sleeping on my bed, usually in the company of one of the cats. During my naps, he'd think nothing of hopping up beside me and stretching out at my side. By the end of the summer, he'd stretch out flat on his tummy under the swing set with my children swinging above him and not so much as a flick of the ear.

Thumper brought joy into our lives with all of his funny ways. When Red Dog died, he was there to ease the hurt. Eleven days after Red Dog's death, I noticed that Thumper's eyes were quite swollen. While waiting for my husband to come home from work so we could go to the vet, I cradled Thumper in my arms. He started to cry and very soon I could tell that my comical fat friend had died. It was horrible. Nevertheless, I rushed to the emergency vet, but it was true. Thumper was really gone.

I buried Thumper myself next to Red Dog. For a very long time afterward, the back yard that had once been so full of happy memories had become an empty place to me. I hated to go there.

What can I say to you, but that I still feel the loss and I am crying now as I write about my two friends. But at least, I guess, one thing that makes me happy is that I had 13 wonderful years with my dog and the privilege of having a white and gray rabbit who could always make me smile.

Thank you for listening and letting me share my words. I know this is a long letter, but I cannot put the love and sadness that I feel in anything less. These animals were so special to me that I had to tell you about them.

K.F., Kentucky

Helping Children with Death

Dear Kymberly,

I am an only child and I was raised with a standard male collie. I learned to walk while holding onto his rear end. I remember being told that he would periodically poke his nose in my crib to check on me. He was my best friend and the closest thing I had to a brother.

My collie died when I was 10 and I still remember the hurt. We buried him on the farm, but I was not allowed to be there — I was told to stay in the house. We never discussed the death or the pain I felt. I cried at school for weeks, but was too embarrassed to tell my teachers that I was crying because my dog had died.

I begged for a new dog. It took almost a year before we found another collie. He was still alive when I married and left home. When my husband married me, he became a kind of father to my collie's son, Shad.

Before long, Shad had a son, which made us a two-collie family. My husband and I added a human son for the dogs to raise. I was beginning to feel threatened by all these males, so we added a female collie pup. In time, I gave birth to another son. Our family was complete — two beautiful sons for our three collies to raise.

As all responsible animal owners know, there comes a time when heart-breaking decisions have to be made. My sons were eight and three when Shad had to be put to sleep. We decided that even though this was clearly a family affair, it deserved as much dignity and honor as if it were being conducted in a public place. My husband and I have always raised our children in total honest reality. We were also concerned with the fact that this was the first time our children would be confronted with what DEAD really means.

The whole family — my husband and I and our two sons, then three and eight years old — buried Shad. My youngest son understood what was going on. He knew what "put to sleep" meant and he saw Shad's body wrapped in a plastic bag.

Together, we selected a special place in the back yard. We each took one turn with the shovel to dig the grave and then cover it up. All of us cried hard as we did this. We talked about all the things — wonderful and bad — that had happened to us because of our dogs. We talked about Heaven, Jesus and that just because you can't see someone, it doesn't mean they aren't alive in your heart. We buried the dog with his own bowl, his favorite candy bar and lots of love.

We have buried two more pets in the last seven years and, unfortunately, we will probably bury another soon. We have followed the same ceremony because it helps us and we find comfort in it.

We had a neighbor child staying with us when our last crisis happened. He cried along with us and still talks about Dancer's funeral. His parents think we are crazy, but were not offended by our actions. The child doesn't understand why, when a pet dies at his house, it isn't a big deal.

My children have been spared the loneliness of not having a pet after one had died, but they have learned that all animals have special personalities and cannot be replaced with substitutes. They have also seen firsthand how animals grieve for one another.

We must all face the reality of death and I feel it is really important to give children the chance to see that this is so. I hope that by helping our children understand that death is something that happens, whether we like it or not, and by exposing them to our methods of dealing with hurtful losses, we have given them the tools needed to deal successfully with the future.

Sincerely,

D.P., Oklahoma

Appendix

The Spiritual Dimension

Introduction

Many of the letter writers made references to the spiritual dimension as they struggled to come to terms with the loss of their animal companions. Because I share their interest and concern, I wanted to learn more about what our great religious traditions — Western and Eastern — have had to say about this often overlooked part of God's creation. At the same time, however, I realized that humanists too, despite their lack of belief in a divine plan, might have given some thought to the subject of death as a phenomenon of nature that touches all creatures.

It is hard to imagine that any animal lover who believes in an afterlife for humans has not also thought seriously about the implications of that belief for his beloved pet. I have encountered many people who simply cannot imagine a heaven without the presence of the animals with whom they shared their lives.

When I began to look into the spiritual place of animals in the traditions and sacred writings of the world's great religions, I was surprised to find that there were more references than one might think, given the almost total lack of discussion of the topic in modern-day life. Many readers are no doubt aware of the great love of St. Francis for animals of every kind, but less well known is the deep attachment that the Prophet Muhammad had for his animal companions and his concern for their welfare in the next world.

One important discovery I made was that while all the major religions have concerned themselves with the humane treatment of animals as an important part of the life and right conduct of believers, not all of them explicitly address the question of whether there is an afterlife for animals. But even in the case of those faiths that do not offer an answer to this question, one clear belief emerges: God's love for animals is undeniable, and His love must mean that they are always under His care.

In this section I have attempted to take a look at the place that animals hold in the religious traditions of the West and the East, as well as the unique perspective offered by humanism. I conclude the section with a selection of extracts from the letters of some of the writers who responded to my appeal, in which they speak of their own beliefs about a spiritual dimension that extends to their beloved animal companions.

Western Thoughts

The writings of Judaism, the wellspring of Western religion, declare that everything created of God is holy and that nature and animals are part of the good things in life. This idea is illustrated by a prayer recorded in the Mishnah, the collection of Jewish traditions that became the basic part of the Talmud. It was intended to be said by an observant Jew at the sight of a beautiful animal:

> Blessed art Thou, O Lord our God, King of the Universe, Who hast such things as these in Thy world.

The following comment has been attributed to the great rabbi and teacher, Sherira Gaon, who lived in tenth-century Baghdad. Rabbi Gaon was speaking about the slaughter of animals for food, and although this is not the specific subject we are addressing here, it is in this passage that reference is made to the value and honor to be accorded to animals in the divine plan. The phrases "due reward" and "just recompense" as used in this passage suggest that the worth and suffering of animals are indeed noted by the Creator. Rabbi Gaon clearly believed that there is a plan for animals, that they have not been forgotten:

> ...but the Creator did not deprive the animals of a due reward, and we may believe that all creatures...will be rewarded for their pains, for there is no doubt that God the Holy One does not deny just recompense to any of His creatures. In this

sense the animal has, therefore, not been created in order that evil should be inflicted upon it, but in order that good should be done to it; nor is it by any means created for the purpose of being slaughtered, although this has been permitted to man.[1]

THE OLD TESTAMENT

The Old Testament, regarded as sacred scripture by Jews, Christians and Muslims, includes many positive references to animals, their importance and their unique identity. The book of Ecclesiastes (4:19-22) contains these significant lines:

> For that which befalleth the sons of man befalleth beasts; even one thing befalleth them; as one dieth, so dieth the other. Yea, they have all one breath; so that a man hath no preeminence above a beast; for all is vanity. All unto one place; all are of dust, and all turn to dust again. Who knoweth the spirit of man that goest upward, and the spirit of the beast that goest downward to the earth?

The writer of Ecclesiastes is asking the question that we ask today when we have lost our animals. Who is to say that upon death only humans go "upward"? Among those of us who have shared our lives with animals, some would certainly agree that to suggest that only humans go "upward" is indeed "vanity."

Nearly everyone is familiar with the story of Noah's ark in the book of Genesis in which the close interaction of humans, animals and God is magnificently portrayed. Noah and the animals obeyed the personally given orders of God. Noah built the ark and the animals came in pairs of their own accord, without his needing to fetch them. Later, when the Great Flood subsided, the cherished Covenant between God and humanity was established (Genesis 9:9-17). God promised never again to destroy the world by flood, and in the promise He included "every living creature." Chapter 20 of the book of Exodus records how God delivered the Ten Commandments to Moses. The Fourth Commandment, "Remember the Sabbath day to keep it holy," is interpreted to mean that on the seventh day work should cease. The need for rest on the Sabbath was intended not only for humans, but also for draft animals (Exodus 20:10; Exodus 23:12; Deuteronomy 5:14). God's plan took into account the exhaustion of cattle after pulling a plow for six days. This concern reappears later in the New Testament, where the watering of cattle on the Sabbath is approved (Luke 13:15). Again, humans and animals are meant to share a place in the divine code of life.

Man's responsibility to the animals around him is illustrated in many scriptural passages: in Exodus 23:4, where the just are enjoined to lead straying oxen to safety; in the very next verse, where animals struggling under too heavy a load are to have their burden removed; in Deuteronomy 22:10, where plowing with an ox and an ass yoked together is prohibited so that the stronger ox could not bring hurt to the weaker ass; in Numbers 22:23, where the Angel rebuked Balaam for beating his ass.

Many scholars agree that numerous passages scattered through the Old Testament show a concern for the welfare of animals and a compassion for their needs that were far in advance of anything written until the nineteenth century.[2] An interesting example is the injunction of Moses not to muzzle oxen even if they trampled on the corn growing in the fields (Deuteronomy 25:4). Moses and David were considered ready for leadership only after they had proved themselves as shepherds; in Old Testament times, men were not permitted to buy animals unless they could show that they could properly provide for them. And it was considered wrong for a man to eat his meal before he had fed his animals.[3]

Psalm 148 calls upon all of God's creatures to praise Him and give thanks. The Psalmist mentions angels, kings, princes, maidens and children, but he also includes the great sea creatures, the beasts of the field, all creeping things and flying fowl — all of these created by the same God.

Proverbs 12:10 reinforces the idea that animals are part of God's plan for human conduct when it states, "A righteous man regardeth the life of his animals."[4] Drawing upon the Old Testament teachings regarding the proper treatment of animals, modern rabbis have held that it is legitimate to grieve for a departed pet and to treat that pet's remains with tenderness and respect. At the same time, however, mourning that exceeds the bounds of a reasonable reaction to a death serves to impede the mourner's ability to carry on normally with his life.[5]

THE NEW TESTAMENT

The story of the birth, life, death and resurrection of Jesus is the focal point of the New Testament. Jesus began his teaching ministry at the age of 30. His words were recorded by his followers.

In Mark 7:14, Jesus says, "All of you listen, and try to understand. Your souls are not harmed by what you eat, but by what you think and say." And Jesus gives an example in the story of the Syro-Phoenician woman (Mark 7:25-30):

> Right away a woman came to him whose little girl was possessed by a demon. She had heard about Jesus and now she came and fell at his feet, and pled with him to release her child from the demon's control.
>
> Jesus told her, "It isn't right to take the children's food and throw it to the dogs."
>
> She replied, "That's true, sir, but even the puppies under the table are given some scraps from the children's plates."
>
> "Good!" Jesus said. "You have answered well — so well that I have healed your little girl. Go home, the demon has left her!"

The account of this exchange in the fifteenth chapter of Matthew has been interpreted to refer to a dog that was domesticated and considered part of the household.[6] It is commonly believed that dogs were the first animals that were taken as companions, with evidence back to the late Stone Age. In the Near East of biblical times, however, the practice was far less common, with dogs considered scavengers by some Old Testament writers. The cat, first domesticated and later deified by the ancient Egyptians, was long associated with pagan ritual by the Hebrews.

In I Corinthians 15:35-45, the resurrection of the dead is discussed:

> But someone may ask, "How are the dead raised? With what kind of body will they come?" How foolish! What you sow does not come to life unless it dies. When you sow, you do not plant the body that will be, but just a seed, perhaps of wheat or of something else. But God gives it a body as He has determined, and to each kind of seed He gives its own body. All flesh is not the same: Men have one kind of flesh, animals have another, birds another and fish another. There are also heavenly bodies and there are earthly bodies; but the splendor of the heavenly bodies is another. The sun has one kind of splendor, the moon another and the stars another; and star differs from star in splendor. So will it be with the resurrection of the dead. The body that is sown is perishable, it is raised imperishable; it is sown in dishonor, it is raised in glory; it is sown in weakness, it is raised in power; it is sown a natural body, it is raised a spiritual body. If there is a natural body, there is also a spiritual body.[7]

The Catholic writer and Trappist monk, Thomas Merton, had this to say about the relationship of God to all creation:

> The only true joy on earth is to escape from the prison of our own false self, and enter by love into union with the Life Who dwells and sings within the essence of every creature and in the core of our own souls.[8]

One popular belief concerning St. Francis of Assisi is that he frequently offered prayers for sick and dying animals. He is also thought to have believed that in God's infinite love all things were possible and that prayers for all His creatures — including those beyond earthly life — were a natural part of the charity expected of the faithful.

THE QUR'AN

The Qur'an (sometimes also spelled Koran) speaks to every aspect of a Muslim's life. As the final revelation of Allah to the Prophet Muhammad, it gives specific instructions on such things as marriage, divorce, social responsibility and the religious practices required of believers. The authority of the Qur'an is believed to be absolute. The chapters, or surahs, of the Qur'an (indicated here within quotation marks) contain many references to the love of Allah for animals.

> He created the beasts which provide you with warm clothing, food and other benefits. How pleasant they look when you bring them home and when you lead them out to pasture! They carry your burdens to far-off lands, which you could not otherwise reach except with painful toil ("The Bee," 16:1).

The Qur'an states that it is not necessary for the faithful to practice animal sacrifice. Allah doesn't need animals to die for Him to know what is truly in a believer's heart ("The Table," 5:101).

> No one dies unless Allah permits. The term of every life is fixed ("The Imrans," 3:142).

Of particular significance is this passage:

> All the beasts that roam the earth and all the birds that wing their flight are communities like your own. We have left out nothing in Our Book. They shall all be gathered before their Lord ("The Cattle," 6:36).[9]

The Prophet Muhammad expanded on this idea:

> All God's creatures are His family; and he is the most beloved of God who doeth most good to God's creatures."[10]

Muhammad was once asked if there were rewards for doing good to four-legged animals, such as giving them water to drink. Muhammad answered:

> Verily, there are heavenly rewards for any act of kindness to a live animal.[11]

Muhammad's affection and respect for animals can be seen in stories passed down through many generations of Muslims. One popular story concerns his relationship with a cat. Once while in the midst of prayer, Muhammad interrupted his sacred ritual to give water to his thirsty cat. On another occasion, as Muhammad began to prepare for prayer, he noticed that the cat had curled up on his robe. He then cut the robe in such a manner as not to disturb the cat and silently moved away. Yet another story records that one of Muhammad's companions was so fond of cats that he became known as Abu-Khurairha, or "Father of Cats." Abu-Khurairha is believed to have inquired of the Prophet whether cats might find their way to Paradise. Muhammad considered the question and replied, according to some accounts, that not only cats but also dogs and horses could show merit during their earthly lives and so earn a place as companions to the faithful in the Garden of Paradise.[12] In Muslim mystical tradition, a bird whose call accompanied a true believer at prayer might also find a place in the world to come. This tradition is particularly associated with the nightingale, but the love of Allah for the songs of birds is alluded to in several respected sources.[13]

The mystics of Islam are known as Sufis, or "men of wool," so called because they originally wore woolen robes. The wool was sheared only after asking the consent of the animal providing it. The following poem, by the well-known Sufi poet Jelaluddin Rumi, is called "The Long Journey":

> I died as a mineral and became a plant,
> I died as a plant and rose to an animal,
> I died as an animal and I was a man.
> Yet once more I shall die as a man,
> To soar with angels blest;
> But even from angelhood I must pass on:
> All except God doth perish.[14]

NOTES

1. Sherira Gaon Defends the Rights of Animals, in Franz Kobler (ed.), *Letters of a Jew Through the Ages*, vol. 1 (New York: Schocken Books, 1980), p. 121. This source was made available to the author by the kind assistance of Roberta Kalechofsky of Jews for Animal Rights.
2. *New Bible Dictionary*, 2nd Ed. (Wheaton, IL: Tyndale House, 1982), pp. 40-41.
3. Wallace Sife, *The Loss of a Pet* (New York: Howell Book House, 1993), p. 138.
4. *The Holy Bible, New King James Version* (Nashville, TN: Thomas Nelson, 1979).
5. Sife, *The Loss of a Pet*, pp. 139-140.
6. *New Bible Dictionary*, p. 41.
7. *The Guideposts Parallel Bible* (Grand Rapids, MI: Zondervan, 1981).
8. Philip Novak, *The World's Wisdom* (San Francisco: HarperCollins, 1994), p. 276.
9. *The Koran*, translated by N.J. Dawood (London: Penguin, 1956).
10. Philip Novak, *The World's Wisdom*, p. 315.
11. Ibid., p. 319.
12. R.A.C. Crofts-Young, *The Oral Tradition in Islam* (London: Unwin, 1924), p. 408.
13. Ibid., pp. 409-410.
14. Novak, *The World's Wisdom*, pp. 328-329.

Eastern Thoughts

HINDUISM

In Hindu thought, our present state is the net result of our past deeds, our karma. To advance, we must make the best use of the body and mind we are given, whether in the form of an insect, a fish, a bird or a mammal. The ancient Hindu text known as the *Padma Purana* stated that there are 8,400,000 species of living things and each individual being (called a jiva) must experience each of them. A jiva reaches the human form after spending many centuries as other life forms. Respect for these life forms helps to explain the widespread practice of vegetarianism among Hindus. As one advances, the responsibility that must be taken for one's actions is increased. The temptation of worldly desires lessens steadily as one progresses. As the learning process continues, one's "karma dues" diminish.[1]

    Although the learning part, or soul, is individual, it does not proceed alone. It always carries within itself a part of the Omnipresent or Godhead. In Hinduism, this Godhead does not possess a personality. God permeates everything, with creation waxing and waning depending on the cycle, never beginning and never ending. After passing through the human incarnation, bodily death can bring the soul into a state of connectedness with God. Whether individuality survives death is not certain. The thread of individuality runs through Hindu thought, but not all Hindus agree on its definition. But for all Hindus, advancing toward bliss means flowing in and with God.[2]

Gandhi, the great Indian philosopher and leader, believed that compassion for animals had been allowed to grow lax with the breakdown of spiritual devotion in India, especially during the long period of British rule. In this respect he reflected the views of the religious Jains of his native Gujarat, who rejected all aspects of animal sacrifice and held that even the smallest creatures must be protected from harm of any kind. It is for this reason that some Jain monks and nuns wear a cloth covering over their mouths to prevent the accidental inhalation of a flying insect. Gandhi was particularly concerned that an eroding compassion for cows and other hard-working animals had led to a decline in the morality of modern Indian society. It is for this reason that he strongly advocated the enactment of strict animal protection laws.[3]

The doctrine of reincarnation ties all creatures to each other. As a result, respect for animals of every kind conveys an essential respect for their souls as they progress through each succeeding incarnation. In this respect, no distinction is made between wild and household animals except in the sense that the latter may be in closer proximity to assuming human form, though this remains a debatable assumption.

The *Bhagavad Gita* ("The Song of the Blessed One"), the most widely read and loved of Indian classics, contains a passage that truly embodies the Hindu view of death and earthly loss:

> ...he who dwells in the body is eternal and can never be slain. Therefore, you need not grieve for any creature.

BUDDHISM

The founder of what we now know as Buddhism was a young Indian prince named Siddhartha Gautama. It was not only the sight of human suffering that disturbed his heart, but the suffering of animals, too. He observed that both men and oxen were overworked and treated callously, and he decided to seek the answer to why there was so much pain in the world.

When Siddhartha decided to set off to find the Way, going on a journey called the Great Renunciation, he chose to take his beloved horse, Kanthaka. As he made ready to leave, he turned to his horse and said, "O brave one in fight and fearless, put forth strength as in a stern battle, for tonight I ride far to seek deliverance not for men only but for your kind also."

When they came to their journey's end after a very long trip, he thanked Kanthaka for a job well done. When the horse was to be returned home, Siddhartha said his final goodbye: "My horse, gentle and noble, your good deeds have gained their reward. No painful rebirth awaits you, this I know. Be content, for it is well."[4]

Devout Buddhists refuse to take any life or offer sacrifices of blood. This example was set for them by Siddhartha when, having achieved Buddhahood, he stepped in to save goats who were about to be sacrificed by Brahmin priests. The priest who was about to begin the ritual was beseeched by Buddha to spare their lives. In this respect, Buddha departed from the Hindu reverence for animals that disallows consumption as food while reserving certain animals for sacrifice to a god. Because of its unique standing with the gods, the cow is regarded as inviolable in all respects. But Buddha took the position that like humans, animals are trying to find the Way and must be allowed to make their life's journey without violent interruptions. He is said to have remembered his own previous incarnations as various animals and often fashioned his parables around them.

The compassion and deep respect for animals shown by Siddhartha throughout his life were carried through his teachings into many lands beyond the borders of India. In Thailand the adoption of Buddhism more than a thousand years ago entailed a special new role for a special breed of cat. Respect for the intelligence and bravery of the cat led to the appearance of the highly revered temple guardian cats who were the ancestors of the modern-day Siamese. Not since the ancient Egyptians had cats been treated with such deference and solicitude. The well-developed and diversified vocal sounds of the Siamese were regarded as ideally suited both to warn monks of danger and to frighten away intruders. So esteemed were these guardian cats that their care was entrusted to only the most favored monks and they were permitted a diet of the choicest fish, foods limited to major feast days for the rest of the population.[5]

Buddhism differs from Hinduism regarding the concept of the soul. Buddha did not believe that living beings had a tangible, individual soul. When one attains liberation from the cycle of life and death, this victory is an opening to the passionless peace of Nirvana. Nirvana is not a heaven with a personal god, as one might conceive of a higher state in Western thought. For the Buddhist, Nirvana is a blending or a becoming of all that is. No individualism or self-conscious thought exists any longer. Complete freedom, melding, enfoldment and expansion are but a few of the gifts of Nirvana. There are no words, in any language, to adequately define and explain Nirvana; it is simply a place of complete belonging. Thus the notion that animals would be forever excluded from this higher state would be unthinkable in both traditions. From the accounts we have to go by, it appears that Kanthaka attained Nirvana without so much as passing through the human form.

The offering of prayers for animals that have died is not only allowed but often encouraged in Buddhist practice. It is not unusual for prayers and devotional passages to be read aloud to household pets for their possible edification. Buddhists believe that it can be beneficial for an animal to be exposed to religious art and family rituals. Such exposure is thought to be an aid to the animal in securing a favorable future incarnation. Beginning on the day of the companion's death and continuing as a part of a family's daily devotions, the offering of a short prayer dedicated by name to the departed animal is a practice reported among Tibetan Buddhists and also found among the devout of Thailand and Burma.[6]

NOTES

1. M.J. Stutley, A *Dictionary of Hinduism* (Oxford: Oxford University Press, 1977), pp. 84, 116, 236, 297.
2. Zaehner, R.C., *Hinduism* (Cambridge, MA: Harvard University Press, 1970), pp. 12, 18, 24, 29, 67.
3. Geoffrey Parrinder (ed.), *World Religions: From Ancient History to the Present* (New York: Facts on File, 1971), pp. 237-238, 240, 241.
4. L. Adams Beck, *The Story of Oriental Philosophy* (New York: Farrar and Rinehart, 1928), pp. 128-129.
5. D.R. Feingold, *A Social History of Theraveda Buddhism* (Hong Kong: University of Hong Kong Press, 1984), pp. 97-98, 117, 124, 136.
6. Wallace Sife, *The Loss of a Pet* (New York: Howell Book House, 1993), pp. 145-146; Feingold, *A Social History of Theraveda Buddhism*, pp. 137-138.

The Humanist Perspective

There are many who do not identify with the thought of a God or an afterlife. Some may feel more comfortable with the rationality of natural law to guide them through the death of a loved one. The philosophy of humanism embraces this view of life and its end.

Corliss Lamont, an American philanthropist and the author of *The Philosophy of Humanism,* gave what is probably the most succinct explanation of the humanist view of death:

> The death of anyone whom we love, no matter what his age, stabs deep into the heart and leaves a lasting pang.[1]
>
> ...Humanists look death in the face with honesty, with dignity and with calm, recognizing that the tragedy it represents is inherent in the great gift of life.[2]
>
> ...I must add that it is by no means so terrible a thing as many religions and philosophies have depicted. If the humanists are right in calling immortality a brain-woven conceit, death not only does away with the possibility of an eternal paradise, but also negates the threat of hells and purgatories beyond the tomb. Death destroys unjustified fears as well as unjustified hopes. Since a man can die only once, the dead are beyond all good or ill. They are as totally unconcerned with life and existence as the unborn and unconceived.[3]
>
> ...Death in and of itself, as a phenomenon of Nature, is not an evil. There is nothing mysterious about death, nothing supernatural about it, that could legitimately lead to the

interpretation that it is a divine punishment inflicted upon men and other living creatures. On the contrary death is an altogether natural thing and has played a useful and necessary role in the long course of biological evolution.[4]

UNITARIAN UNIVERSALISM

Although not all Unitarian Universalists regard themselves as strictly humanist (in that they do not choose to deny absolutely the existence of a God and a life after death), they do consider themselves as essentially tied to the earthly plane.[5] Nevertheless, Unitarian Universalists affirm the inherent worth of all creatures. Because animals share our world with us, they are deserving of honor and compassionate treatment. Therefore, when animal companions die, their loss is both real and significant.[6]

Unitarian Universalists consider it appropriate to mourn the death of a pet as a sign of love and respect as well as a means of taking leave of a valued companion. Part of this leave-taking is acknowledging the loss and another is remembering all the happy times that were shared with a beloved animal friend.[7]

NOTES

1. Corliss Lamont, *The Philosophy of Humanism* (New York: Continuum, 1949), pp. 105-106.
2. Ibid., p. 106.
3. Ibid.
4. Ibid., p. 102.
5. Christopher Jay Johnson and Marsha G. McGee (eds.), *How Different Religions View Death and Afterlife* (Philadelphia: The Charles Press, 1991), pp. 297-298.
6. Ibid., pp. 300-303.
7. Wallace Sife, *The Loss of a Pet* (New York: Howell Book House, 1993), pp. 143-144.

Thoughts from the Letter Writers

"And this much I truly believe: when my time comes to pass over, their dear faces will be the first ones I see and no one will ever be able to separate us again."

A.D., New York

"It's been one and a half years since Holly went to Heaven. We read lots of books on different religions searching for answers and we know she's sitting right by the gate with her little shiny eyes and perky ears just waiting."

M.N. and I.N., Washington

"I know she is in heaven, looking down, remembering all the wonderful times we had."

A.K., California

"I believe that our pets wait for us in heaven and that he will be there when I get there to greet me at the door."

J.B., Iowa

"I received sympathy cards from Amber's doctors and from friends. One that stands out showed paw prints on the beach and a ball laying in the sand. Inside it said, 'Your friend has gone on ahead to wait for you.' I believe she has and that someday we will be together again. The idea that animals do not have souls is to me ridiculous!"

L.L., California

"There is a 'flower chart' hanging on the inner door of the church that I attend. It's the custom for parishioners to sign their names under a particular Sunday they would like a friend or loved one honored or remembered, and donate the altar flowers on that day. I check out the month of April and find the second Sunday is open, sign my name and add, 'In Memory of a Friend.' It doesn't matter, really, that our members won't know who my friend was, or more specifically, that it was my German shepherd, April, who would have been 12 years old on April eighth. It just matters to me that on her birthday she'll be remembered. Then, I scratch through the words 'In Memory of a Friend.' I write, 'In Memory of April.' I close my eyes and I can see her. And it occurs to me that wherever she is now, she knows I am remembering. I swear she knows!"

N.C., Maryland

"When I pass to the beyond, I was told by a man of the cloth that my dog will be waiting for me. He told me dogs have souls, all living things do and there is room in heaven for us all. I pray to see my beloved Hobo. He was a very big part of my life and I'll love him forever and ever."

C.H., Tennessee

"You can only begin to know how deep the heartache of this experience of loss is when you experience it personally. The fact is, when you lose a husband, parent or child, you know where their soul goes — back home to be with God. That's what the minister says, it's in the Bible and you have hope. You ask, 'Is my dog with God too? Is she running free, no longer in pain, and happy in Heaven?' When you ask these questions, you are looked at as if you are no longer responsible for your thoughts. The last answer you want to hear is, 'Well, the Bible does not state for sure that dogs have souls nor where they go when they die.' What kind of theological training did ministers receive when they can't answer a simple question, 'Is my dog with God?'

"Let me tell you, Mi Girl had a soul. In my heart I know. It was a beautiful soul. Often I think God sent her to me as an angel, then took her back when he needed her more than I. In retrospect, if loyalty and a beautiful spirit count for anything, then I know dogs go to Heaven. That's where Mi Girl is, and I pray someday to see my best friend and companion again."

B.S., Iowa

"We hurt so badly because we loved Chalk so very much. We just wanted to share these verses with you.

"Psalm 34:18: 'The Lord is near to the broken-hearted, and saves those who are crushed in spirit.'

"Revelations 21:4: 'And He shall wipe away every tear from their eyes; and there shall no longer be any death; there shall no longer be any mourning, or crying, or pain.'"

M.M. and D.M, Texas

"Molly's death was two days after Christmas, and the neighbors came over to console me: 'Molly has gone up with Baby Jesus. He needs a good watchdog.' I retired her leash and collar, put away her food and water dish, but she is everywhere, gone to a land of lush grass, to run forever unleashed."

G.G., Ohio

"I believe that someday God, in His mercy, will allow me to be with Tribble and all others I have loved, in a world where there is no disease or pain. I cling to that hope."

Author unknown

"As a Christian, I would like to envision Jesus meeting me someday in heaven. Beside Him would be my beloved parents, and in His arms, my Dupus. 'Here is your pet,' He would say, smiling. Just to envision that possibility fills my eyes with tears and my heart with hope."

L.V., New York

"I've often thought that God did make one mistake in creation — not giving us pets that live as long as we do."

D.R., Vermont

"I pray to God and ask Him to let Wishbone sit in His lap every once in awhile and maybe 'dance' with him and give him a window to sit in so he can look out over the world."

K.S., Oklahoma

"I prayed for his spirit and soul, each day, to be released and allowed to be free to go where it must now be. Snowflake, be strong, and one day, if it's possible, our spirits will be interlocked again. Until then, Snowflake, I miss you and deeply love you."

P.Y., California

"Another thing that makes it easier is that I know I will see her again someday. I am sure she is in heaven. She will be there waiting for me."

S.S., California

"I do have comfort in knowing that Boo is with my parents in heaven and that they are taking care of each other until I get there."

J.D., Texas

"To us, Wendy is not gone but in heaven and we will see her one day."

L.C., Texas

"I just hope that she will forgive and/or understand my making this very difficult decision for her and hopefully 'all dogs do go to Heaven.' I, for one, definitely want her waiting on my doorstep in my 'mansion in the sky.'"

M.B., Kansas

"One of my biggest problems still is finding the right terminology for explaining the loss of my dog. I have been saying that Schroeder 'went to doggy heaven' because it makes me feel better to think that he's in a 'good place' (I'm trying to be a 'good person' so we can be together when we're both gone!)."

L.B., New York

"I told Rocky, while I was saying goodbye to him, that I was quite certain what he would see and hear and feel at the moment he was set free: light, beauty, new life, freedom from pain. And that he would have a job — He would be a protecting angel.... He was a guardian. I think he still is, even now.

"People who think animals do not have souls are arrogant, selfish, smug and stupid. I know animals do. And I also know that Rocky has been with me since his death. Not always, but I think he just needed to make sure that all would be well."

K.H., Washington

"I only hope that dogs go to heaven because when I die I expect to see my dogs waiting for me. If they aren't, then heaven doesn't exist."

C.G., Pennsylvania

"I know that this may sound silly, maybe even sacrilegious, but in my heart, mind, body and soul, I know that somehow, some way, God will allow me to see and be with my precious Melli again someday."

M.J.K., California

"When God created the animals, He intended for them to live forever...the Spirit of God that would have sustained us and the animals for all eternity, without the interruption of death, is the same Spirit that will resurrect all creation when Jesus comes back.

"Dear Friend, never allow anyone to intimidate you because you care about animals. Concern for the eternal destiny of one's pet is as much a part of pet ownership as anything else. It is interesting that Proverbs 12:10 reads: 'A righteous man regardeth the life of his beast....' It could have said 'the welfare of his beast;' but God chose the world 'life,' and I believe, again, this is characteristic of His nature: He is concerned with life.... In Proverbs 12:10, the Amplified Bible adds the world 'consistently' in brackets: 'A [consistently] righteous man regards the life of his beast....' So caring about animals is consistent with righteousness. God Himself is always consistent: If He asks us to care about animals, He has designed that relationship to be eternal. God does not abandon that which He has created. Nor is he a wasteful God: He would not create a life to have it come to nothing in the end."

Frances Arnetta
Christians Helping Animals and People, Inc.
P.O. Box 272, Selden, NY 11784

Helpful Resources

If you would like to seek additional sources of comfort, support and information, the material in this section may be helpful. This is a very basic listing of some online addresses, books, hotlines and places to write for advice and assistance on coping with the loss of a companion animal.

ONLINE SITES AND SERVICES

There is an enormous amount of information regarding this topic on the Internet and I recommend that readers take a look. The following is a listing of sites that I feel are worthwhile:

American Veterinary Medical Association (AVMA)
http://www.avma.org

The "Care for Pets" portion of this site contains an excellent section on pet loss and euthanasia. There is also a listing of grief resources for adults and children, as well as phone numbers for pet loss grief support hotlines.

alt.support.grief.pet-loss (Pet Loss Newsgroup)

A newsgroup devoted solely to the topic of grief resulting from the loss of an animal companion. People may post stories or messages, ask questions and read what other people have to say about their experiences with this type of grief.

The International Association of Pet Cemeteries — Death of a Family Pet
http://www.aros.net/~petcem/grief.html

This site gives information about the stages of grief and euthanasia of companion animals. Also included is advice on choosing a burial site for your pet, suggestions for planning a burial ceremony and a list of veterinary colleges that offer pet loss support services.

The Virtual Pet Cemetery
http://www.lavamind.com/pet.html

A very popular site where pet owners may literally create a virtual gravesite for their departed animal companions. Many gravesites include poems, stories or epitaphs. In addition, The Virtual Pet Cemetery publishes an online newsletter and supports a bookstore solely devoted to pet-related books.

Pet Grief Support Page & Candle Ceremony
http://petloss.com

A self-proclaimed "gentle and compassionate" website for pet lovers who are grieving over the death or illness of a pet. Offers support and advice and hosts a candle ceremony every Monday night. People may post a request to have their special thoughts about their pet remembered in the next candle ceremony and they can also list the pet's name. In addition, this site contains links to a number of grief resource pages and lists the phone numbers of telephone support hotlines.

Pet Loss: A Reference to References
www.superdog.com/petloss.html

A superb site for information and links to books, audiotapes, resources, memorial items, cemeteries and hotlines. Each link is annotated so you can more easily find what you are looking for. The book reference section recommends books about pet loss for adults and children, and even lists one that addresses the grief that animals feel when they've lost a fellow animal friend.

Rainbow Bridge
http://www.primenet.com/~meggie/bridge.html

The Rainbow Bridge page is a place where grieving individuals may post tributes to pets that have passed on. Visited by many, many people, this site also includes an online chat room where people can receive support from others who have or are experiencing the grief that comes with the death of a beloved pet.

BOOKS

Animals: Our Return to Wholeness
Penelope Smith. Pegasus Publications, 1993. 351 pages

This book addresses the spirituality of animals and our relationships with them. There are chapters discussing the death and reincarnation of animals. There are stories of communication with all living beings, including birds, cats, dogs, snakes, whales and many more. A beautifully inspiring and uplifting book.

Bless All Thy Creatures, Lord: Prayers for Animals
Edited by Richard Newman. Macmillan, 1982. 130 pages

A one-of-a-kind book that offers prayers for animals (including birds, fish, farm animals, dogs and wild animals). There are also prayers for people who have lost animal companions, and prayers for children to say and learn. A touching and beautiful anthology.

Coping with the Loss of a Pet
C.M. Lemieux. Wallace R. Clark Publisher, 1988. 50 pages

A short but helpful book for those who are hurting from the loss of a pet. Examines the experience of grieving, sadness, anger and guilt and offers advice on how to cope with these feelings. Small and light enough to carry with you should you find that you need words of comfort while at work, or any place.

Other Creations: Rediscovering the Spirituality of Animals
Christopher Manes. Doubleday, 1997. 288 pages

A unique book that traces the history of writings about animals in religious literature.

Pet Loss: A Spiritual Guide
Eleanor Harris. Llewellyn Publications, 1997. 258 pages

This book explores the timeless love and connection between people and their pets. The author discusses the stages of grief and offers guidance through meditation and ceremonies to help heal the pain.

Pet Loss: A Thoughtful Guide for Adults and Children
Herbert Neiburg and Arlene Fischer. Harper Perennial Library, 1996. 151 pages

An excellent book that acknowledges the pain felt by people who have lost animal companions and offers advice on coping with the anguish. Includes sections on the sudden death of animals, helping children to deal with their pain, and the loss of a pet by means other than death.

The Souls of Animals
Gary Kowalski. Stillpoint Publishing, 1991. 114 pages

A book on animal spirituality that addresses the emotions of animals and their awareness of loss. An excellent source for learning how to help an animal who has lost a companion.

ORGANIZATIONS

Censhare
P.O. Box 734, Mayo Memorial Building
420 Delaware Street, SE
Minneapolis, MN 55455
(612) 624-5909 (leave message)

The Center to Study Human-Animal Relationships and Environments (Censhare) is dedicated to improving and investigating the bond between animals and humans. A valuable clearinghouse of information, including books, newsletters and videotapes on pet loss.

Delta Society
289 Perimeter Road East
Renton, WA 98055-1329
(800) 869-6898 (voice); (800) 809-2714 (TDD)
(425) 235-1076 (fax)
http:/petsforum.com/deltasociety/dsn100.html

An excellent resource for information and references on grief and pet loss. The Delta Society has a directory of counselors who specialize in grief from pet loss. They also offer brochures, videos, bibliographies and other helpful aids.

HOTLINES

Please note that the hours and phone numbers listed below are subject to change.

Chicago Veterinary Medical Association
(708) 603-3994
Phone is always open for voicemail messages, but calls are only returned between 7 and 9 pm (Central time). This line is monitored by veterinarians. Note that long-distance calls are returned "collect."

Michigan State University Veterinary Clinic
(517) 432-2696
Staffed by veterinary students from Tuesday through Thursday, 6:30 to 9:30 pm (Eastern time).

National Mental Health Hotline
(800) 969-6642
A clearinghouse for information on bereavement, grief, loss, depression, and other problems a person may experience. Number is toll-free and open 24 hours a day.

Ohio State University School of Veterinary Medicine
(614) 292-1823
Support hotline is open on Monday, Wednesday and Friday, 6:30 to 9:30 pm (Central time).

Tufts University School of Veterinary Medicine
(508) 839-7966
Hotline is open Tuesday and Thursday, 6 to 9 pm (Eastern time) and is staffed by students. During off hours, students will some-

times respond to voicemail messages.

University of California, Davis, School of Veterinary Medicine
(916) 752-4200
Manned by veterinary students, this is one of the more well-known hotlines on pet loss. Open weekdays from 6:30 to 9:30 pm (Pacific time).

University of Florida School of Veterinary Medicine
(904) 392-4700
Veterinary students monitor the phones during the hours of 7 to 9 pm (Eastern time).

Virginia-Maryland Regional College of Veterinary Medicine
(540) 231-8038
Phone lines are open Tuesday and Thursday from 6 to 9 pm (Eastern time).